Zen Heart

Simple Advice for
Living with Mindfulness
and Compassion

EZRA BAYDA

Shambhala
Boston & London, 2008

SHAMBHALA PUBLICATIONS, INC.
Horticultural Hall
300 Massachusetts Avenue
Boston, Massachusetts 02115
www.shambhala.com

9 8 7 6 5 4 3 2 1

FIRST EDITION

Printed in the United States of America

⊛ This edition is printed on acid-free paper that meets the American National Standards Institute Z39.48 Standard.

Distributed in the United States by Random House, Inc., and in Canada by Random House of Canada Ltd

Library of Congress Cataloging-in-Publication Data
Bayda, Ezra.
Zen heart: simple advice for living with mindfulness and compassion/Ezra Bayda.
p. cm.
ISBN 978-1-59030-543-0 (hardcover: alk. paper)
1. Spiritual life—Zen Buddhism. 2. Zen Buddhism—Doctrines. I. Title.
BQ9288.B399 2008
294.3'444—dc22
2007041862

Contents

Contents

Part Three
Cultivating Being Kindness

Zen Heart

What Is Our Life About?

Our aspiration, our calling, our desire for a genuine life,
is to see the truth of who we really are—
that the nature of our Being is connectedness and love,
not the illusion of a separate self to which our suffering clings.
It is from this awareness that Life can flow through us;
the Unconditioned manifesting freely as our conditioned body.

And what is the path?
To learn to reside in whatever Life presents.
To learn to attend to all of those things
that block the flow of a more open life;
and to see them as the very path of awakening—
all of the constructs, the identities,
the holding back, the protections,
all of the fears, the self-judgments, the blame—
all that separates us from letting Life be.

And what is the path?
To turn away from constantly seeking comfort
and from trying to avoid pain.
To open to the willingness to just be,
in this very moment,
exactly as it is.
No longer so ready to be caught

in the relentlessly spinning mind.
Practice is about awakening to the true Self;
no one special to be, nowhere to go.
Residing in the Heart, just Being.

We are so much more than just this body,
just this personal drama.
As we cling to our fear,
and our shame, and our suffering,
we forsake the gratitude of living from our natural Being.

So where, *in this very moment*, do we cling to our views?

Softening around the mind's incessant judgment,
we can awaken the heart that seeks to be awakened.

And when the veil of separation rises,
Life simply unfolds as it will.
No longer caught in the self-centered dream,
we can give ourselves to others,
like a white bird in the snow.

Time is fleeting.
Don't hold back.
Appreciate this precious Life.

—An earlier version of this poem appeared in
Being Zen: Bringing Meditation to Life

Introduction

The Three Phases of Spiritual Practice

WHEN I FIRST began spiritual practice, my single driving goal was to become free from the discomfort of anxiety and fear. I firmly believed that if I made intense efforts to go against my fears, I could eventually overcome them and be rid of them. I also had the deeply held belief that with one single enlightened experience, my life would be forever clarified.

Since then, and particularly since I became a Zen teacher, I have seen countless students begin practice with similar illusions. Such illusions are based on the hope that one magical experience will change us forevermore, or that somewhere there is a formula capable of unfolding the mysteries of spiritual practice. The problem is there are no shortcuts. It's not that practice is so terribly complex; it's more that practice cannot be reduced to a simplistic or instantaneous solution to life's difficulties.

Nonetheless, we can still talk about what spiritual practice is and what it isn't. *Practice* is a term that is hard to define. In a general sense, the term is synonymous with "spiritual path." For example, saying we have a Buddhist practice means we are following the spiritual path of the Buddhist tradition. But we can also talk about practice in a more concrete way, such as when we refer to specific techniques like meditation practice or prayer practice. Perhaps the most common way the term *practice* is used is to describe a particular type of effort, one associated with trying to live a more awake and genuine life. When we

3

refer to "practicing with daily life," or "practicing with emotions," we are using the term in this way, which includes all the ideas and techniques that focus on the effort to *practice* maintaining awareness.

Over my years of practicing and teaching Zen, I have found that there are three somewhat distinct and essential phases in practice; and the purpose of this book is to clarify how these three phases interweave to allow the wonder of awakening. Whether we are beginners or have been practicing for many years, our ongoing task is to clarify and deepen our learning. Dividing practice into three distinct phases can be very helpful in this learning process, by allowing us to better grapple with the sometimes daunting effort to cultivate inner freedom and equanimity.

Why three phases? And why these particular three? Although the terminology may be unfamiliar, each of these three phases describes a particular *inner* process that each of us must go through on our spiritual journey; and while there are no distinct or fixed dividing lines between the three phases, the unique inner process associated with each phase needs to be addressed individually. In fact, when any one of these phases is not explored, or even worse, when it is ignored, as often happens when we follow the path of least resistance, our spiritual maturation may be severely hampered. The point is, in order to have a complete spiritual practice—one that includes awakening in each of these unique but interpenetrating phases—it is helpful to have a clear and straightforward explanation of what each of these phases entails.

The first phase—the Me Phase of practice—involves clarifying all the ways we're run by the self-centered mind. It includes uncovering our most basic beliefs, observing our typical emotional reactions and patterns of behavior, and perhaps most important of all, becoming very familiar with our fears.

This Me Phase was once considered to be more a part of the discipline of psychology than a part of spiritual practice, but it is now widely recognized that we need to know ourselves on a psychological level before we can enter deeply into the other aspects of practice. To "know thyself" has been a pivotal part of most spiritual traditions; here we will be considering it in depth in order to free ourselves from the self-centered drama of "me."

The second phase—the phase of Being Awareness—intensifies as we become less involved with "me" and more concerned with cultivating a larger sense of what life is. Much of what is called "mindfulness" or "sensory-awareness practice" fits into this category, and it's an essential aspect of many spiritual traditions. But as presented in this book, it goes beyond basic awareness of the sensory world to include the transformation of the narrow inner experience of a "me" to a more spacious sense of being.

The third phase—the phase of Being Kindness—has to do with learning to live from the awakened heart. In essence, it's about connecting with the loving-kindness and compassion that are our true nature, and learning to live from that place. This aspect was not directly addressed in the Zen tradition that I was trained in; loving-kindness and compassion were seen as qualities that would come forth naturally on their own as we mature in practice, rather than qualities that needed to be specifically cultivated. And while it is somewhat true that loving-kindness and compassion may flower on their own in the course of a practice life, in many traditions these qualities are seen as indispensable, and are given much more emphasis from the very beginning.

My own experience has made me appreciate the necessity of cultivating Being Kindness directly, as a crucial aspect in deepening and intensifying our spiritual journey. When I was in my late forties, I became seriously ill with a chronic condition of the immune system. For months on end I was so weak and nauseous that I was unable to practice in the way in which I was trained; I couldn't sit crossed-legged in meditation, nor could I focus my mind enough to concentrate. Only after reading Stephen Levine's *Healing Into Life and Death*, where I learned to do the loving-kindness and other heart-oriented meditations, was I able to experience a whole new dimension in practice. Instead of lying in bed in despair, I learned that my suffering could be the direct path to awakening the heart. Until then I had looked down on "heart" practices as being superficial, but now I realized I had been leaving out an extremely valuable and essential aspect of practice.

I prefer the term *Being Kindness* to *loving-kindness*, in part because it helps us bypass the common conception that loving-kindness is about a good feeling. Using the less familiar term *Being Kindness*, we have a chance for a fresh inquiry into the nature of the unconditional friendliness that is at the core of Being Kindness.

Although these three phases often follow in a natural progression, they are not necessarily consecutive. For example, working on the second phase of Being Awareness does not require being completely done with the Me Phase. In fact, the three phases interweave from the very beginning. The spaciousness of Being Awareness and the heart quality of Being Kindness allow the work of the Me Phase to proceed with more compassion and less self-judgmental harshness. The main point is that each of the three phases addresses a different essential aspect of our spiritual development, and depending on where we're at, one phase may require more attention than another.

The Me Phase

The first phase is the clarification of what makes a "me." Unfortunately, many students mistakenly try to jump over the first phase and go directly for the expanded experience of spaciousness that characterizes the latter phases. I mentioned that, when

I first began spiritual practice, my main motivation was to be free from fear. But rather than doing the basic work of the Me Phase, which would necessarily involve bringing awareness directly to the fear, I chose to ignore it and instead focus intently on the breath. I believed that if I practiced long enough and hard enough on cultivating the spaciousness of the breath, the fear would dissolve on its own.

This is problematic, because we can't simply leave our personal conditioning behind. We can't let it go just because we see that it is irrational and getting in the way, or because we want to move on. If the course of spiritual practice were that simple, we'd all be awake right now. The fact is, moving beyond the Me Phase is extremely difficult. Our conditioning goes very deep, often becoming physically rooted in the body. As a consequence, our conditioning has to be addressed directly, at least in part, before we can enter more deeply into the phases of Being Awareness and Being Kindness. It took me several years to realize that trying to bypass the Me-stuff was backfiring, in that whatever we ignore or push away just gets stronger.

The clarification of what makes a "me" is not a philosophical or theoretical inquiry; the work has to be very specific, very empirical. Clarifying our thinking means knowing, with precision, what our actual beliefs are. This does not necessarily involve looking at our past, or analyzing why we think the way we do. Rather, this is an objective process, where we simply notice the present content of the mind. During this phase we learn to use techniques that help us see our thoughts *as* thoughts, and not as The Truth.

Our basic beliefs, or illusions, are like the lens filter on a camera; they color how we interpret and relate to reality. Think for a moment whether you are aware of what your most basic stance toward life is. An example might be "Life is too hard." Now ask yourself what your most basic belief is about yourself. Do you know? It could be something like "I'm basically inadequate," or

"I have to struggle." Clearly seeing our specific beliefs about ourselves is of crucial importance, because so much of our suffering is based on unconsciously holding on to these beliefs without ever questioning their validity. Until we see these beliefs clearly and repeatedly—the beliefs that make up the basic story line of "me"—they will continue to dictate how we feel and act. This is why this first phase of practice is so important, because if we ignore this aspect, we will continue to live from our deep-seated conditioning.

However, the first phase of practice is not limited to simply looking at our beliefs. We also need to become aware of and observe our most frequent emotional reactions. Do you know yours? Is it anger? Anxiety or fear? Confusion? Observing these reactions doesn't require having judgments about them; it only requires seeing our own patterns as clearly as possible.

The same observations can be made about our conditioned strategies of behavior. For example, ask yourself what you most often do once you've been caught in an emotional reaction. Do you withdraw? Attack? Seek escape? Go numb? Do you try to analyze or fix the situation? Again, in spiritual practice, you don't have to try to change anything; the point is only to see as clearly as possible what you do. Yet, it's ironic that when we clearly and repeatedly see what we do, without trying to fix ourselves, transformation comes on its own.

The last and most basic aspect of the first phase of practice relates to our fears. Fear is often at the root of our motivations and behaviors; it affects how we dress, how we talk, and how we act and react. Though sometimes our fears are obvious, most often they remain hidden. Yet it is absolutely fundamental that we learn about our own particular fears. For example, do you know the two or three things you fear most? Do they come to mind readily? If not, this crucial aspect of self-knowledge will have to be explored further in all three phases of practice.

Eventually, in the Me Phase of practice, we have to move from simply observing our emotions and fears to actually entering into them, or residing in them, *experientially*—which means to feel them fully in the body. This is not something most people are used to, and we may have little interest in doing it. Consequently, this is a place where many students get stuck, because they equate residing in an emotion with wallowing in it, a state in which we continue to believe our thoughts or hold tightly to an emotion. Yet the difference between the two is critical. Residing in an emotion occurs when we feel the physical experience *nonconceptually*— that is, without being hooked into the story line of thoughts, the story line of "me." Dropping the story line of "me" is one of the most essential steps on the path to awakening.

For example, if we become angry, it's very easy to wallow in it, continuing to replay thoughts such as "This isn't fair," or "No one should have to put up with this." But when we refrain from entertaining the thoughts, and instead feel the heat and pressure in the body, we move from wallowing to actually residing in the anger. Moreover, truly residing in an emotion means that awareness becomes a bigger container. And in that bigger container of awareness, what was once experienced as the narrowness of "me and my sensations" widens to include the air and surrounding sounds, as well as the visceral experience in the body. When emotions are experienced on this level, rather than remaining tied to thoughts and judgments, they are eventually transformed from something solid and dark to simple energy, which is movable, porous, and light. Paradoxically, it is by paying objective awareness to this small sense of self that we connect with a larger sense of self.

Being Awareness

At this point, we are already moving beyond the Me Phase into the phase of Being Awareness. But please be clear: we're never completely done with the Me Phase; there will always be some little subterranean remnant from the past that still has some juice left in it. However, at some point this aspect becomes less prominent in our practice life, and when emotional reactions do arise, they're seen much more quickly and their duration and intensity are much diminished. As the Me Phase begins to require less attention, we begin to devote more and more of our practice efforts to the phases of Being Awareness and Being Kindness.

Being Awareness is an expanded sense of what life is. Sometimes, to cultivate this, we may need to undertake specific practices, such as paying attention to the breath or to surrounding sounds, which allows us to begin to move beyond the skin boundary of "me." But this second phase of practice also includes simple awareness as we go through our daily life—feeling our feet on the pavement, actually seeing the trees, looking into the eyes of another without our normal agendas. Within these very simple practices there often comes a sense of delight in just *being here*.

Yet, as straightforward as this may sound, we often ignore the importance of this less dramatic, more mundane, aspect of practice. For example, many students mistakenly think that practice is primarily about sitting in meditation in order to feel a particular way, such as calm or spacious, or primarily about working with emotional difficulties, and as a consequence, place much less emphasis on the cultivation of simple awareness in everyday life.

Another common detour away from Being Awareness is actively trying to achieve a more expanded state of consciousness. This is really just more Me-stuff, in that we are still stuck in the self-centered drama of "me," trying to be different. That's why it's so important to focus on the first phase for a long time; in truth, it is the only way to see through the psychological mechanisms that get in the way of living more awake.

Whether we are cultivating Being Awareness through specific meditation practices or through awareness in everyday life, it has one particular defining quality: the sense of "I" begins to change. Instead of our habitual and fixed view of "me," which is held in place by all of our stories, we develop a more fluid view of what this thing we call a "self" really is. As our stories become less solid, when we say "I," there is a knowing that it's not quite the truth of all that we are. Instead, we begin to experience a very particular sense of being, which is the visceral experience of presence. There is a vividness—the quiet texture of simply being.

Right now, bring awareness to the texture of the moment. Feel the breath. Feel the sensations in the body. Now add to that the experience of the room—the spaciousness of the room. And while staying with the experience of the breath and the room, feel the sense of "I am here." Try to stay with this sense of presence for a few breaths so that you can get a taste of what the state of Being Awareness actually is.

When Being Awareness is activated, the sense of "I" does not necessarily disappear, nor does it have to. But it transforms from "I" as "me" to "I" as "Awareness." The I-as-Awareness is not the little or self-centered "I," but rather something quite different. And although it can't really be described, it is more real than anything. It includes a knowing of who we are, which is no longer limited to just our stories or just our bodies.

I-as-Awareness is not about how we feel emotionally. It's not about feeling high or relaxed or calm. How we feel emotionally is still on the level of Me-stuff. Waking up is about awareness, not our state of feeling. Awareness is simply the context in which emotional feelings, pleasant or unpleasant, come and go. As we see through the various aggregates of I-as-a-me, our solid sense of self begins to dismantle, leading to the growth of I-as-Awareness.

I-as-Awareness, or Being Awareness, is not a magical or mystical experience. It is simply the experience of an awake presence. And although in one way it is the natural state of who we are, it does not necessarily come to us naturally. It requires all of the clarification of the Me Phase of practice, as well as an ongoing effort to turn away from mechanicalness and waking sleep, qualities that seem to be almost hardwired in human beings.

But even hard wiring can be transformed. With an ongoing practice of awareness, as the sense of I-as-Awareness grows, so does our ability to be more awake to the texture of life, and to connect with and experience others with appreciation. We will still have difficulties, but our difficulties are no longer so difficult. In fact, at a certain point we may even cease to view them as difficulties, but perhaps instead as opportunities to simply be present to what is. Being Awareness becomes just that—the equanimity of becoming awake to, and resting in, being itself.

Being Kindness

There is no distinct dividing line between the phase of Being Awareness and the phase of Being Kindness, in which we learn to live increasingly from the awakened heart. In fact, even work done in the Me Phase has a distinct impact on the third phase. After all, how could we ever live a life of Being Kindness if we were still totally caught in the self-centered story of "me"? Being Kindness can range from heartfelt friendliness all the way to unobstructed love toward everyone and everything.

It's been said that we can learn to see the face of God in everyone and everything by bringing a gentle awareness to the heart that's still too closed to see. We don't usually hear much about God in Zen, but the "God" in this statement is not the God of religion; it is simply another way of referring to the sense of connectedness, or the ineffable energy of reality that unites all and everything. To see the face of God in everyone and everything is another definition of love. Not personal love, with all the ups and downs of emotion, but the love that is the essential nature of our being. The real problem is that we can't just love simply because we want to. Most of the time, we can't see the face of God in anyone or anything, let alone everyone and everything.

Consider this: right in this moment, can you experience the face of God? Can you experience love? This is not about a warm, fuzzy feeling, or the "I" that loves "you." In experiencing love on this level there is no "I" that loves. This is simply love itself.

Again, there's no point in trying to be loving, because in that very trying we are blinded to the face of God. Trying to be loving, trying to be anything, trying to feel any particular way— whether it be loving, calm, clear, enlightened, healthy, happy, kind, or whatever—is not what waking up to our true nature is about. Waking up is about learning to say "yes" to everything. This doesn't mean passively or indiscriminately saying that everything is okay. Instead, it means we're willing to be open and curious about what our life really is. But how can we say yes when we're so busy pushing away the things, the people, the fears, we don't like? Saying yes requires first and foremost paying attention to the no, the inner contraction we feel toward all that we would like to be different, all that we reject and push away, whether it be in ourselves, in the world, or in another person.

Right now bring to mind one specific person in whom you can't see the face of God, someone whom you can't genuinely appreciate for who he or she is. Do you instead feel anger, resentment, or judgment? What are your strongest beliefs or requirements? If you don't know, ask yourself, "How is that person *supposed* to be?"

These requirements are the illusions that separate us. They are illusions because they're based on fantasies of who the other person is or is not, and on what they can or should be doing for us.

Now, still keeping this person in mind, what is the physical experience in the body? Can you feel the bodily contraction—the physical experience of constricted energy and visceral tightness? Can you see how this contraction, combined with your belief about how the other person should be, is exactly what constitutes the "self"? And furthermore, that this "self" is exactly what prevents us from seeing the face of God in another?

Practice must entail bringing awareness to the sense of "self"—in other words, to the heart that is still too closed to see. This self is not something vague or amorphous. It could take the form of disappointment, or the belief that things will always go badly. The self is exactly this belief of discouragement, as well as the physical feelings in the body that accompany the belief.

When we feel rejection, or lack of appreciation, undoubtedly our bodies will contract, or we will manifest emotion in some physical way. That contraction, that sense of self, is exactly where we must bring awareness. When we feel the anxious quiver in our being, that felt sense that something is wrong—whether it's from the fear of losing control or the feeling that life is unsafe—in that anxious quiver is where the self solidifies.

Practice is about learning to address these painful feelings. Yet we don't address them by trying to get rid of them. Rather, we address them by bringing nonjudgmental awareness to them. The path of Being Kindness, in part, requires bringing our gentle attention to the very things that seem to block our way to it. We don't have to change who we are—our thoughts or our feelings. We just have to be aware of them. Awareness is what heals; this is the one most fundamental tenet of our practice.

Peace—that sense of inner calm we all aspire to find—is not found through striving to attain it. It's found only through residing fully and completely in what is, whether it be the most peaceful or the most tumultuous experience of our life. Only by residing in what is, exactly as it is, will our self-imposed prison walls come down. And when they do, all that remains is the connectedness that we are. All that remains is Being Kindness.

As we learn to reside in what is, as we develop the ability to let our experience just be, we can begin to go deeper into practice. No longer so focused on just working with our stuck places, we can begin to explore the depth to which the specific meditation practices of Being Kindness can take us. Learning to live increasingly from the awakened heart allows us to experience the basic connectedness that we are. It also leads to the growth of compassion for others, particularly as we are freed from our own self-judgments. There is nothing in this life more satisfying than connecting with the Being Kindness that is our true nature and then learning to live from it as the natural response to whatever life presents.

The Me-stuff may always be there, but we can learn to hold it more lightly. Leaving the world of Me-stuff and entering into the unconditional friendliness of the heart connects us with the immediacy and preciousness of life. Even when life appears to be a total mess, on some fundamental level we know it's okay.

A good example of what it looks like to live from the awakened heart of Being Kindness is in the literary figure Larry Darrell, from Somerset Maugham's *The Razor's Edge*. After many years of searching and devoting himself to spiritual practices, Darrell, whose character was based on a real-life person, achieves not only clarity but also a deep connection with the love that is our essential nature. When he returns from his search back to everyday living, it is obvious that he could become a famous spiritual teacher. But instead he chooses to be a cab driver in a big city, where he can simply give to others from his own being, without fanfare or agenda—like a white bird in the snow.

In the second phase of Being Awareness we learn how to maintain a bigger sense of what life is. As we live increasingly from I-as-Awareness, we may come to understand one of the most basic spiritual truths—that all is One. But attaining this truth does not guarantee that we will understand the other most basic spiritual truth—that all is Love. Learning this second truth is the fruit of living increasingly from Being Kindness. There are certainly examples of long-term practitioners, including teachers, who attained wisdom and spaciousness in the phase of Being Awareness but who didn't develop the heart quality that is the essence of the phase of Being Kindness. In a complete practice the spaciousness of Being Awareness will dovetail with the heart quality of Being Kindness, and it is only then that we can say that we are living from the Zen Heart—the truth of who we really are.

The rest of this book concerns how, specifically, to take the three steps toward a complete spiritual practice. I have divided the book into three parts, to reflect these three basic steps. Although there is ample precedent for the division of spiritual practice into three, such as Christianity's trinity or Buddhism's three treasures, I don't claim any particular esoteric basis for my three-part division; rather, this framework is more a practical one. From my many years as a practitioner and a teacher I have observed how a well-balanced practice life needs to develop in these three basic phases or steps. When any one of these steps is ignored, or even downplayed, spiritual development remains short-circuited. The first step, which I call the Me Phase, is becoming free from the attachment to "me." The second step, entering into Being Awareness, is to open up to a much more spacious sense of what life is. And the third step is to learn to live from the Being Kindness that we are.

All along the way there will, of course, be smaller steps. I have divided each of these smaller steps into threes, in part to make them more workable and in part to trick the little mind, which will consider things more readily if they sound simple and within the little mind's control. But don't be fooled. There can never be a simple one-two-three step to freedom.

Nonetheless, as the ancient proverb goes, the journey of a thousand miles must begin with a single step. And then another step. And then another. While each one of us must take these steps on our own, this book will attempt to clearly describe each step along the way. Although I am a Zen teacher, the three phases or steps described here are not tied to one particular tradition or religion; rather the teachings are universal, based on the three inner stages of development that are necessary components of a complete practice. It is my hope that this book will serve as a guide along the path of becoming who we truly are.

PART ONE

The Me Phase of Practice

1
Detours from Reality

ONE OF THE GREATEST HINDRANCES to living a more awake life—a life of satisfaction and appreciation—is that we spend most of our time lost in the mental world. We are literally addicted to our thoughts, whether we are planning, fantasizing, worrying, dramatizing, conversing, or whatever. If we are honest, isn't it true that most of our time is spent spinning in thoughts?

There are three habitual grooves where most of us get caught spinning in the mental world: analyzing, blaming, and fixing. These conditioned patterns are detours from being present to reality, and taking any one of them guarantees that we will perpetuate the story line of "me." In fact, being caught in the mind, whether through analyzing, blaming, or fixing, is one of the prime aspects of the Me Phase of practice.

Analyzing

When a difficult situation arises, one of our first reactions might be to ask why. We analyze the situation by asking, "Why is this happening?" "Why am I depressed?" "Why am I so tired?" "Why am I anxious?" and so on. We ask why, in part, because we want certainty; we want to maintain the illusion that our lives are guided by certainty and logic. We want to avoid the anxious quiver of the present moment, the discomfort of not having ground under our feet. We think that through analysis, we can uncover why we think the way we do, why others are doing what they're doing, or why something happened the way it did. We think this mental understanding is necessary for our comfort. But, most of the time, does asking why on this level give us much real clarity or satisfaction? Don't we usually end up just spinning in circles? Granted, when we uncover our believed thoughts—those repeated thoughts that we have a habit of taking as reality—we can sometimes see how these thoughts impact our emotional reactions, but most often, the reasons we come up with are, at best, only marginally accurate.

I once visited the Catacombs of Paris, where the bones of six million dead bodies are piled neatly along a mile-long corridor, deep beneath the streets. I imagined how many times in the lives of all of these people the question, why is this happening? was asked—the vanity of thinking we can actually figure life out. There was an apt inscription carved in the walls: "Silence, you mortals. Great vanity—silence."

From a practice perspective, the real question is not why but what—what is my life right now? Or even better, *what is this?* This question moves us out of the mental world into the experiential. The question, what is this? is really a Zen koan. The Zen koan is traditionally a question that a teacher gives to a student, but koan-questions cannot be answered with the conceptual or analytical mind. In fact, a koan such as "What is the sound of one hand clapping?" is specifically meant to baffle our normal thinking mind, and in so doing allow us to experience the spaciousness of the nonconceptual. Asking, "What is this?" serves as the perfect koan because, like any koan, there is no way you can answer it by thinking or analyzing. In fact, the only answer to this question is the actual experiencing of the present moment itself. The only answer is "Just this!"

Right now, ask yourself, "What is this?" To answer, simply feel the breath going in and out. Feel the air in the room. Feel the tension in your face. Feel the energy going through your body. Experience a felt sense of the overall body posture. Experience "just this!"—the simple quality or texture of the moment.

Gutei, a ninth-century Zen master, would often respond to students' questions by simply raising his index finger, saying nothing. Instead of getting an answer, students would be forced into being present with their own experience. Can you imagine the frustration of coming to talk to a teacher, expecting the comfort of intellectual clarity or psychological insight, and being met only with silence? However, even if we did find it frustrating, that silence can be an invaluable teacher. Instead of conceptualizing, instead of asking why, students would have to face the "what" of their experience. They could no longer use their thinking to escape what was happening *right now*.

Rather than holding together the "me," we can begin to turn away from the comfort of fixed identities—identities that are held in place by our thoughts. Every time we have a thought about ourselves—"I'm the kind of person who . . ." or "I'm like this because . . ."—we solidify the concept of a "me." On a subtle level, even beliefs such as "I'm a Democrat" or "I'm an American" feed the I-as-a-me. But to see through these artificial mental identities allows us to stop identifying exclusively with the little self, and connect more and more with a larger sense of life—a sense of Being Awareness.

Naturally, when difficulties arise in life, we look for answers, because we prefer the comfort of black-or-white thinking. We continue to hold on to the notion that we can figure life out; yet, the fact is, we'll never figure life out by asking why. Most often, we just don't know.

My mother told me a story about her father at the end of his life. He was a very religious and humble man, well respected in his Orthodox Jewish community. From his sick bed he requested a prayer book so that he could recite the Friday night prayers.

Everyone tried to tell him it was not Friday night, but he persisted in his request. Finally someone got concerned about his seeming lack of clarity and went to ask the rabbi for advice. The rabbi understood that my grandfather knew he was about to die, and told them they should honor his request and gather around him for the prayers, which they did. Shortly after he finished praying, he passed away. The knowing that my grandfather tapped into is not readily accessible to the thinking mind, nor can the mystery of what life is ever be explained by easy formulas or by what we think of as "knowledge."

My wife, Elizabeth, and I recently visited the concentration camps at Auschwitz-Birkenau. The hardest part, much more than the verbal descriptions of the systematic cruelty and horror, was seeing the piles of baby clothes and the photographs of the individual human faces, especially the mothers and children clinging together as they got off the train, not knowing that they would be dead within a few hours. All the lives cut short. The completely arbitrary nature of it. Even the most comprehensive practice overview can't explain or make sense of something like this. Platitudes such as "There is no life or death," or "Within emptiness everything is perfect just as it is," are hollow words, denying the basic fact that within life there is inexplicable suffering. We can do our best to learn from it, but there are no easy solutions, no overarching explanations. The experiential, rather than any mental explanation, is what opens and transforms us—such as seeing the piles of baby clothes and letting the image etch itself into our hearts.

Even to look for profound spiritual wisdom may be a detour; much of what passes for profundity may be just confusion that's well stated. To accept that we really know very little may be uncomfortable, but it will certainly bring us back to this basic fact: that only through returning again and again to the "what" of our experience itself—the physical experience of what our life is right now—can we enter into and live from the nonconceptual understanding that is the basic essence of our being. Like it or not, it is exactly where we must go if we wish to stop our attempted escapes and detours from what is real.

Blaming

The second equally fruitless detour is blaming. We continually fall into the trap of looking for someone to blame. Some of us may be very aware of this pattern, while for others, it is so subtle or hidden that we don't even realize we are doing it. Either way, blaming has a very compelling quality; it has a certain juice or power, almost like an addiction. Yet, justifying ourselves and blaming others can keep us spinning in the mental world for hours, days, or even years. But if we look closely enough, we'll see that blaming is primarily a defense against feeling the anxious quiver of our own experience.

For example, say we're criticized and have an emotional reaction such as hurt. It's very likely that past hurts will reinforce our present feelings, and our reaction may hit us much more deeply than the present situation warrants. But in order to avoid feeling the painful emotional reaction, we immediately move into the defensive strategy of blaming and self-justifying. We defend so that we don't have to feel the pain of unworthiness or rejection that the criticism triggers. In blaming, we focus on the perceived faults of the other, to detour away from having to direct our attention inward, which we fear might be extremely uncomfortable.

The practice countermeasure to blame is to directly face the pain we are trying to avoid. This is not a mental process; it involves feeling the pain, residing in it, as the *physical* reality of our life. I'm talking about doing something very straightforward, yet very difficult, which is to cut through the story line of blame and instead stay in the present moment of our experience. We simply don't want to do that. Yet, this is where the sense of separateness, of the "me-ness," transforms into Being Awareness.

To enter the present moment of hurt, ask yourself what that hurt actually feels like physically. Remember, the word *hurt* is just a concept. Although as a mental concept it may seem very complicated or overwhelming, as an actual physical experience in the body it becomes very specific. Again, we're back to the koan-question "What is this?" Is there an ache in the heart, queasiness in the belly, or an overall heaviness or rawness in the body?

Whatever you experience when you feel hurt, or any other emotion, the practice is always to bring awareness to the energy coursing through the body, rather than thinking or analyzing. If thoughts arise, notice them, but rather than getting caught in the story of me, especially the story of blame, keep awareness focused on what is felt in the body. You could also include awareness of sounds, or other aspects of the environment outside of the skin boundary—this will help keep the experience from becoming too narrowly focused on "me and my body."

Please be clear that I'm not talking about wallowing in our feelings, which is what we usually do when we believe all our thoughts about being wronged. Instead, I am describing how to actually feel—fully feel—the physical reality of the present moment. With awareness our suffering becomes more porous, and the energy of life can naturally flow through us. Refraining from the mental fixation of blaming is an absolute prerequisite to experiencing the sense of connectedness that we truly are. Blaming always separates; it always disconnects. In fact, when we're caught in blaming, the sense of "me-ness" is never more solid.

Fixing

The third major detour is fixing. When a problem arises, we almost automatically ask, "How can I fix it?" We instinctively feel the need to find the safety and comfort that come from taking whatever is "wrong" away.

What do you usually do when a difficulty arises? Think about this for a moment. Look at your own patterns. Is your strategy, for example, to withdraw or close down in order to avoid dealing with hardship? Or perhaps you have a more aggressive strategy, such as meeting your difficulty head-on in order to take care of it right away. Or maybe your strategy is to worry obsessively, or to bury yourself in diversions. We can even use meditation as an escape, by trying to bypass our problems with an artificial sense of calm.

All of us need to become aware of our own strategy of escape, our own specific patterns of trying to "fix" our experiences. It's a given that we don't want to feel discomfort, but since it's inevitable, we have to learn how to address it. This is the blue-collar work of practice, and an integral part of the Me Phase of practice. It's not particularly exciting, but is inwardly intense nonetheless. That's why the quality of perseverance is of key importance, because we have to learn to just *stay*, even when our experience is not pleasing us in the ordinary sense. Put simply, the solution is never about fixing, but rather about staying—especially staying with the fear of helplessness and the loss of control.

Here's a small mundane example. One day on a recent trip overseas, Elizabeth and I knew that the next day we had a lot of connections to make, between a boat ride, a bus ride, a train ride, and two flights. We also had a lot of luggage, so I knew the logistics would be difficult. That night I woke up and my mind started going over the scenarios for the next day. Feeling anxiety, my mind went right to the question, how can I fix this? The answers that came back were pretty much surface thoughts, such as, "Maybe we should take a cab instead of a bus" or "Maybe we should ship some luggage."

This question about how to fix the situation was not necessarily an escape, because on an objective level something could certainly be done to make the trip less complicated. However, the real issue was that the question, how can I fix this? took on an emotional urgency. This urgency turned what could have been an objective approach to simplifying logistical problems on the trip into an attempt to avoid facing the fear of the loss of control. My practice in this situation was to see clearly where I was caught in the believed thoughts of dread, and to then stay present with the visceral experience of anxiety. As always, the practice is to stay with the "what," the physicality, of our present moment experience.

We all have experiences like this on a regular basis, where we get caught in the three major detours, asking, "*Why* is this happening?" "Who can I *blame?*" "How can I *fix it?*" We need to watch ourselves take these three escapes time and again, and see if we understand how to implement the practice countermeasure in our differing situations. Again, the countermeasure is "just this"—raising the question, what is this? in order to cultivate a willing curiosity toward the immediacy of our experience. A large part of the struggle of the Me Phase of practice is in turning away from the pull of the three mental detours, and instead staying with the physicality and possible discomfort of our experience.

Even though staying present with our discomfort is counter-intuitive—that is, it goes against our natural instinct for comfort and safety—it is ultimately the only path that offers real freedom. That we will detour off this path by spinning in the mental world is a given. Yet, such detours offer no real escape from our sense of anxiety and unease. Residing in the anxiety, without trying to fix or change the situation, is always difficult, but it also provides a potentially fruitful learning opportunity. Our difficulties can mold us, and our biggest difficulties—the ones we want to avoid the most—offer us the greatest opportunity to break through the protected cocoon of a separate "me." Only by opening directly to our experience itself will we ever tap into the sense of connectedness that is the essence of who we are.

2
Inner Hindrances

THERE ARE THREE HINDRANCES, all of which are ingrained human traits, that keep us disconnected from ourselves: laziness, self-deception, and self-judgment. Like the three detours mentioned in the previous chapter, they diminish awareness of reality. Each hindering trait solidifies the sense of a separate "me," and consequently needs to be addressed in the Me Phase of practice.

Laziness

We rarely use the term *laziness* in talking about practice, because in many ways, spiritual practitioners are often quite disciplined. In fact, the type of effort required in sitting meditation, and particularly at meditation retreats, seems to be the exact opposite of laziness. Yet, we can be very busy and very productive and still be quite lazy—lazy in the sense that we don't want to exert our minds.

For example, a student might come to retreat after retreat but still say with pride, "I don't think about practice," as if thinking about practice is somehow inferior. Yet, it requires some reflection, at least occasionally, to have a clear view of what practice is. Those who are not inclined to think about practice—and this is one aspect of what I'm calling laziness of mind—are often the most confused students, even if they've been sitting for many years. Thoughtful reflection on what practice requires helps keep practice straightforward, and much more possible to actually do. I'm not talking about analyzing our subjective states, but about considering objectively how best to approach practice.

I often suggest to students that they write out a sentence or two on what they see as the point of practice, and to say it each time they are about to sit in meditation. A lot of students resist doing this. Why? Because it requires a definite mental effort to articulate their aim in a clear way. But the benefit of this practice is that it not only gives you a clearer view of what you're doing, it also increases aspiration. What you are repeating each time you sit down to meditate are words you've chosen, words that are particularly meaningful to you.

Of course, to formulate your aim in this way can become very small and self-oriented, but it doesn't have to. Instead, it can be similar to the vows that are repeated regularly at most spiritual centers, words that remind us of the bigger view. For example, at Zen Center San Diego, we recite the following verse at the end of each evening sitting:

> Caught in the self-centered dream, only suffering;
> Holding to self-centered thoughts, exactly the dream;
> Each moment, life as it is, the only teacher;
> Being just this moment, compassion's way.

Even though the bigger view is ultimately a mystery that eludes any precise verbal formulation, we can still make the effort to clarify concepts that point toward the nonconceptual.

Another example of the value of using our minds to understand practice can be observed in working with emotions. For instance, in working with anger, one of the most basic practice principles is to not express our anger. Yet, to follow this dictate without understanding the process would just lead to the unhealthy result of suppressing our feelings. More specifically, we need to understand that only by withholding the expression of anger, that is, by refraining from replaying the story line of thoughts and justifications that accompany it, can we ever move to the next stage, which is to fully feel the anger as sheer energy. Further, we need to understand that anger is often like the mushroom cloud of an explosion, where what is actually at ground zero is the energy of fear. If we don't think clearly about this, if we are lazy in bringing awareness and clear thinking to the process, it becomes much more difficult to go to the heart of the matter.

The point is not to develop into well-trained students who simply follow all the teachings blindly and do whatever a teacher says. You can't let teachers do your thinking for you. Nor can teachers simply rely on practice formulas; teachers also must continually reflect on what practice really is. A good teacher constantly looks for new ways to approach practice, and also continuously probes into what works best.

For example, at a recent retreat, I took a day when we were all practicing complete silence to do a continuous heart practice. The focus was to keep my attention on the breath in and out of the center of the chest while silently saying the words of the Being Kindness meditation. But I knew from prior efforts that resistance would surely arise, so I wrote down four aphorisms on a piece of paper, and every time I lost my sense of purpose, I read one of the aphorisms to bring me back. This is an example of using the mind to bring you back to what is most important.

Another area where laziness of mind often sidetracks our efforts is in self-observation, specifically in observing our thoughts. Probably all of us could stand to be more disciplined and more precise in observing our minds, especially when we're caught in an emotional reaction. Once we get caught in that reaction, it's very easy for strongly held thoughts to pass by unnoticed. That's why one of the most helpful tools is to ask, "What is my most believed thought?" If we don't ask, and if we don't look deeper, how can we ever see through our pretenses and self-images? The reason I'm stressing this point is that our beliefs and conditioned patterns can run unbelievably deep.

My mom, who was eighty-seven at the time and in a lot of pain, and who was also quite aware that she had a very short time left to live, still didn't want to ask the nurse for morphine because she didn't want the nurse to think she was a "dope addict." I would hope that this poignant example could remind us how strong our own self-images are, and how often we're not even aware to what extent they're running our life.

Only by looking deeper—and I don't mean analyzing, but by making an effort that goes against our mental laziness—can we begin to see the beliefs that control us. This kind of effort requires purpose or intention, the intention not to let our repeating emotional patterns just slide by, but instead to look until we see the patterns clearly.

In this vein, the opposite of laziness of mind is inquisitiveness. When a practice idea arises, even while reading a book like this one, we are often too lazy to reflect, or to raise questions. This can indicate a certain dullness of mind, a complacency, a lack of interest in exploring deeper, that prevents us from having a clearer understanding of what we're doing. Or we may settle for easy formulaic answers, characterized by black-or-white, yes-or-no thinking. Of course, it's much easier to imagine we know something than to actually study it. But that's also a guarantee that we won't see through the subtleties of the forces of waking sleep. Only by realizing the magnitude of sleep, and seeing its impact in terms of the harm we do to ourselves and others, will we begin to approach practice with more interest, more effort, more purposeful intention.

The point of seeing through our laziness of mind is not to judge or feel badly about ourselves, but to understand the need to use our minds in the service of waking up. Whether we're thinking clearly about the point of practice, or using our minds to think clearly about working with emotions, or bringing more precision to our self-observations, in every case we need to overcome the lazy tendency to avoid exerting ourselves. There are other ways of looking at things beyond our habitual ones. We don't need to settle for the complacency of what is familiar.

Self-deception

It can be said that regular psychology helps us see what makes us tick, but spiritual practice helps us see that what makes us tick isn't us. In fact, spiritual psychology could be called the psychology of self-deception, in that what we think makes us tick is often a lie. The question is, what are the stories we tell ourselves, the illusions we live out of?

One illusion is that we are in control, or that we *can* be in control. In spite of all the evidence to the contrary, we still live our day-to-day life with the illusion that we're in the driver's seat. And the reason we hold on so tightly to this illusion is that the fear of loss of control is one of our strongest fears.

If you don't think this applies to you, please look again. Look at all of your subtle control strategies. You will most likely find that they are all geared to make your life comfortable and safe, and that they are all based on the illusion that you can, in fact, be in control. For example, we think if we follow the control strategy of trying harder, we can make life go as we would like. Or we might think that following the control strategy of trying to please others will keep us safe from disapproval. Often if takes repeated disappointments in pursuing these control strategies for us to realize that our beliefs of imagined control are in fact illusions.

Another related illusion is the belief that what we "know" is the truth. We believe our perceptions, our opinions, our concepts— forgetting that they are relative, flawed, and limited. In a way, this illusion is a corollary to the illusion of control, in that our imagined "certainty" provides the comfort of believing we're in control. For example, something happens, and we begin asking, "Why is this happening?" We think we can figure things out, and then find comfort in our so-called knowledge. But what we're really doing is holding tightly to the illusion that what we know is the real truth, or at the very least, that we can ultimately figure out what we don't know.

Another universal illusion is that if we practice long enough and hard enough, we'll get what we want—whether it's enlightenment, calmness, freedom from fear, good health, a satisfying relationship, or whatever we're seeking. In the 1960s, like many of my peers, I got caught up in the idea of instant and permanent enlightenment promised in the book *Three Pillars of Zen*. But even if we see through this obvious illusion, this doesn't prevent it from resurfacing later in more subtle forms. You can be sure that this illusion is still on board if you believe that experiencing difficulties or distress means there's something wrong, or even more specifically, that there's something wrong with *you*. This persistent belief, which drives us to do whatever we can to alleviate discomfort, is based on the deep-seated illusion that if we practice hard, we'll feel better. We should never underestimate the extent to which we equate feeling better with being more awake. This is one of the more subtle "lies" we tell ourselves.

In order to live a more awake life, it is absolutely necessary that we drop these illusions. But in order to drop them, we first have to see them. This is why, in the Me Phase of practice, we must repeatedly observe ourselves—the thoughts, patterns, and self-images we take ourselves to be. We must observe our thoughts with precision, so that we'll eventually see that our thoughts, no matter how deeply believed, are not necessarily the truth. It's very common to believe our own illusions, to think we "know" something that is really only a belief. This is why we also ask the practice question, "What is my most believed thought right now?" so that we can go deep enough to uncover the illusions that are normally so hard to see.

Along with these universal illusions—that we're in control, that we know the truth, and that if we do the right thing, we'll get the cookie—there are our individual persona lies, the self-images that we cling to. For example, we could have the belief that we're needy: "I need someone to take care of me, to save me." Or, "I can't be happy if I'm alone." Then there's the pernicious and widespread persona illusion, "I can't be happy if I'm in discomfort." Avoidance of discomfort is one of the most powerful drives in us, yet much of its power derives from the belief—the false belief—that we can't be happy if we're uncomfortable. One of the great benefits of practice is learning that this belief is not, in fact, an unalterable truth.

There are many individual lies or illusions we tell ourselves, and they are as varied as our personalities. For example, do you see yourself as nice, as helpful, as deep? Think for a moment—what is the positive self-image that you cherish the most? Or, do you see yourself more in terms of a negative self-image, such as weak, or stupid, or inferior? Interestingly, we can simultaneously have both positive and negative variants on board and not even see their inconsistency. This is due to the fact that we all wear blinders—a psychological defense that doesn't allow one part of ourselves to see another part. For example, if we need to see ourselves as nice, we may ignore all of our harmful or aggressive qualities. Or, if we need to see ourselves as held back, we'll ignore all the positive data.

Once, in the early part of my practice, I was at a group meeting where we were all having lunch together. The group was based, in part, on the principle of living off the earth, and we tried to grow or harvest all of our own food. As I sat there watching one of the members eat an orange, I was filled with self-righteousness.

I thought, "How dare she not only buy an orange at the store but also have the nerve to flaunt it in a public meeting?" Then I suddenly noticed that I myself was sitting there eating a banana! I immediately felt a sense of shame at my hypocrisy, but I also realized how humorous it was that I could be so self-righteous and simultaneously so self-indulgent, without even being aware of who I was taking myself to be.

This story illustrates another deep-seated illusion: that we are one solid, permanent self. When we see that we are really a collection of many "I's," which are often not even in touch with one another, we realize that this single solid self, this sense of "I," is obviously an illusion. In fact, the whole notion that who we are is limited to a "self" contained by boundaries is perhaps the main illusion that Zen practice addresses.

The difficulty is that sometimes we simply don't want to give up our illusions. There's a story of a father who was trying to get his son to go to school. The son said, "There are two good reasons why I don't want to go: first, it's very boring; and second, the kids always make fun of me." To which the father replied, "There are two reasons why you have to go to school: first, you're forty-five years old; and second, you're the teacher." This humorous story points out how easy it is to lose sight of the things that are central to our lives. What does it take for each of us to stay attuned to what is most important? If we don't know the extent to which we are caught in the self-centered dream of Me-stuff, and if we won't acknowledge that, for the most part, we don't *want* to wake up from our illusions, how will we ever find the equanimity that we seek? How will we ever be open to the truth?

There's a crucial point in practice at which we come to see ourselves in all of our aspects—our laziness, our unkindness, our weakness, all of it. This often comes as a sudden insight, and it can be very sobering. We may feel a sense of shame, but this is different from guilt, which is based on false mental ideals. And it also differs from our normal psychological or ego-based shame, which says, "I am bad."

The shame that I'm referring to is more akin to remorse—it arises when we become acutely aware that we are going against our true nature, against the heart that seeks to awaken. We can feel the pain we cause others, as well as ourselves. When this pain is honestly experienced, it can foster a profound desire to live more awake, more genuinely. From the pain of deep humiliation—from honestly seeing ourselves in all of our waking sleep and in how we go against our true nature—real humility can awaken.

Recently I was sitting on a bench overlooking the ocean doing the loving-kindness meditation. A woman who appeared to be homeless came over to talk to me, but after a minute or so I told her I was busy meditating. Right after she went away, I felt the shock of existential remorse—remorse that came from seeing I was so caught up in meditating on loving-kindness that I couldn't extend it when the opportunity was right in front of me. This was not guilt, but the experience of disconnect from the heart. Allowing ourselves to truly feel this, to take it in without self-blame, is transformative. But the prerequisite to such transformation involves uncovering the self-deceptions out of which we normally live. Seeing through our thoughts, our illusions, our self-images, gradually allows us to enter more deeply into practice. From there, practice moves beyond psychology into a more fluid view of what this thing we call a self really is. When we no longer hold so strongly to our beliefs and judgments, when we don't cling so tightly to our cherished self-images, then, when we say "I," there is a knowing that it's not quite the whole truth. This is where we can begin to experience the clarity of an empty mind—because the mind is not so full of a sense of self, a sense of "me."

Remember, it's awareness that heals. Awareness does not require thinking, analyzing, or judging—just clear, honest seeing. This includes seeing through the more subtle lies we tell ourselves: the lie that we're worthless, the lie that life should be free from discomfort and pain, the lie that teachers can save us, the lie that other people should fulfill our so-called needs.

To enter practice on this deeper level requires, more than anything, a relentless honesty with ourselves. It also requires the willingness to stay present with whatever we're experiencing, regardless of how we feel about it. It's bound to be uncomfortable, because when we first see through our self-deceptions, it's often very painful. Staying in this place requires resisting the urge to move away from our discomfort, the endless ways we try to feel better. It requires the courage, in the poet W. H. Auden's words, to "climb the cross of the moment and watch our illusions die."

Once our illusions start to die, so does the pain of holding on to them. You could say that practice then moves from the heaviness of self-deception to the lightness of just being—of living not from the heaviness of the mind but from the lightness of the Zen Heart. But again, for this to happen, we first have to see through the illusions that normally blind us.

Self-judgment

A critical aspect of the Me Phase of practice is the cultivation of self-knowledge. This means getting to know ourselves in an objective way. When we don't know ourselves—particularly when we aren't aware of the judgments from which we live—we will surely inflict pain on both ourselves and others. Perhaps one of the most basic judgments that causes much of our suffering is the belief in our own unworthiness. This negative self-judgment is deeply embedded in everyone I have ever gotten to know, without exception.

Our deep-seated self-judgments arise early on from the inevitable disappointments of our formative years. Over time, these judgments become more and more deeply ingrained, until eventually, they become what we believe to be The Truth. Until we begin work in the Me Phase of practice, these negative, painfully demeaning self-judgments will not even be open to question.

For example, the deeply embedded judgment "I am unworthy" may not be on the surface of our thoughts, and may even be covered by self-confidence. Yet, because we don't want to feel the pain of this belief, it may nevertheless determine much of how we feel and act. For some, a fundamental belief in their unworthiness may drive them to be productive or to succeed in order to compensate for this sense of inner lack. Others may withdraw or cease trying in order to avoid risking failure. In both cases, the motivation is the same: we don't want to feel the pain of believing we're not enough.

But self-judgment is not just found in our deeply buried self-debasing beliefs. Sometimes our merciless self-judgments are on the conscious, surface level as well, almost as an ongoing frame of mind. For some, it's like having a built-in inner critic who never gives good reviews. If we do something a little silly, the critic is right on board letting us know about it. This can even happen during meditation. How many times have you judged yourself a bad meditator simply because you were daydreaming?

In my beginning years of practice, my self-judgment was relentless. I truly believed in the starry-eyed ideal that if I were a good meditator, my mind would automatically become calm and that I would have special experiences. An expectation like this, however, is a guarantee not only for ongoing disappointment but also for unending self-criticism.

If you remember nothing else, always remember this one great secret of spiritual practice: we don't have to feel *any* particular way. We don't have to have special experiences. Nor do we have to *be* any particular way. With whatever arises, whether it's pleasing or not, try to remember that all we can do is experience and work with whatever our life is, right now. No matter what life is and no matter how we feel about it, all that matters in practice is whether we can honestly acknowledge what is going on, and then stay present with the physical experience of that moment. This is the way we come to experience true appreciation for our lives.

But what is the one thing that most prevents this type of appreciation? Isn't it our deep-seated tendency to judge ourselves as lacking? Self-judgment adds a whole extra layer of suffering on top of whatever pain we might already be feeling.

Buddha told a story about a man who was shot in the chest with an arrow. The pain was great, but Buddha pointed out how much greater the pain would be if the man was shot with a second arrow in the exact same spot. Buddha's point was that we may already feel the pain of disappointment, but by adding the second arrow of self-judgment on top of it, the initial pain deepens into excessive and often unnecessary suffering. For example, if I say something unkind to someone, I will almost immediately feel the pain of being disconnected. But if I add the self-judgment of how unkind I am on top of that, I will feel that much worse.

The countermeasure to self-judgment is always to move out of the mental world and into the physical reality of what is actually present. Self-judgments are always based in thoughts, as either ideals, expectations, or self-images. Such thought-based pictures are always at least one step removed from what is real. Conversely, coming back to what is, even if it's not particularly pleasant, is always a step toward freedom.

I spoke earlier of my initial experiences in meditation, when I would be regularly disappointed by my spinning mind and then judge myself relentlessly (as relentlessly as my mind would spin). Now, many years later, there are still times when I sit down to meditate where my mind is all over the map. However, the difference now is that I am not particularly disappointed, nor do I judge myself as lacking. Instead, I just ride the wave of what is, which in this case is simply scattered energy. To really stay with scattered energy without judgment can actually bring a sense of equanimity.

In order to free ourselves from self-judgment, we first have to be aware of it, particularly how pervasive it is. The more we can see this pernicious pattern with some objectivity, the less we will identify with it as the truth of who we are. This is the work of the Me Phase of practice.

Then, as we increasingly bring awareness to the reality of what is—whether it be the breath, the sounds, the air—we can move beyond the narrow mental world of self-judgment into the more spacious container of Being Awareness. And as an ongoing adjunct to this process, we need to cultivate the attitude of Being Kindness toward our incessant tendency to judge ourselves. To be able to relate to the judging mind with the warmth and friendliness of Being Kindness is perhaps the single most potent antidote to our deeply rooted tendency to judge ourselves.

3

Strategies of Control

JUST AS THE FOOD WE EAT can either nourish or pollute the body, our experiences can also either nourish or deplete our spiritual being. Whenever we engage in self-centered thoughts or actions, we are feeding the growth of our little self, the I-as-a-me; conversely, our conscious life-centered actions help feed Being Awareness, or I-as-Awareness.

"Bad" food, or experiences that we engage in without awareness, also often drain us and leave us depleted of energy for practice efforts. Perfect examples of this are our strategies of control, such as trying to prove ourselves or trying to please everyone. When we play out these strategies, we are usually so caught up in them that we are living in the ultimate self-absorption, and the energy it takes to maintain them often leaves us feeling drained. At the same time we remain full of anxiety.

Here is the essence of the problem: as humans, we have an innate craving for safety, security, and comfort. As a consequence, we develop our strategies of control early on in order to ensure that these cravings are met. But because these strategies become so dominant, our lives begin to narrow, and we are increasingly disconnected from our true nature, our naturally open heart. The energy necessary to awaken is thus squandered by trying to maintain the illusion of control. Yet, no matter how hard we try to maintain our illusions, aren't we all just one doctor's visit away from the total loss of control? Nonetheless,

43

because these strategies often afford at least some form of temporary relief, we remain on the treadmill of our strategies until we realize, at times too late, that we're running on empty.

There are three common strategies of control—trying harder, seeking approval, and escaping/numbing. Some may have only one or two, yet many people have all three.

Trying Harder

When we start with a basic fear such as not being good enough, it makes sense that we would develop a strategy of behavior to counter this. One such strategy is trying harder. For example, the basic belief may be, "If I try hard enough to prove myself, I won't have to feel worthless." So we work very hard to be productive, to demonstrate our value, to excel in whatever we do. We may not even be aware how driven we are by the core fear of being unworthy. In fact, the need to bolster and maintain the self-image of success can be so strong that we may fool ourselves for a lifetime.

Sometimes the strategy of trying harder takes the form of being perpetually busy, or making ourselves indispensable. But still, at bottom, we're trying to validate our own worth. We're desperately trying to avoid the underlying fear of not measuring up. The problem is that no amount of success is enough, because the underlying fear remains unaddressed. Meanwhile, we continue feeding the little self, the I-as-a-me, making it more and more solid. We often make excuses for our busyness by blaming the hectic pace of modern life, but being busy is actually a choice, a strategy of control.

On a subtle level, the strategy of trying harder leaves us with the underlying feeling of restlessness, unable to do the simplest, yet most valuable thing, which is to reside in the moment and feel at home there. The need to *do* something, to be active, is so strong that for many people, the simple act of sitting still, with nowhere to go and nothing to do, is the most frightening thing. The fear that arises—from the felt sense of an inner lack—can range from anxiety all the way to full-blown panic. Ironically, learning to stay with this sense of lack, with the frightening feeling of being no one special, is how we ultimately learn to see through it. There is a very deep satisfaction born of being able to occupy a space without an agenda—to enjoy the inner equanimity of just being, however and wherever we find ourselves.

Realistically, it's possible that the compulsion to try harder, to prove ourselves, may linger for many years no matter how much we work with it in spiritual practice. It may appear again and again in forms that are not so easy to recognize. There was a period a few years ago where I felt very stuck in my practice. Even though I was still quite disciplined, and was doing many of the useful techniques I had learned over the years, I couldn't seem to contact the vitality that I was used to in my practice. It was only after looking deeply at my own believed thoughts that I saw I was caught in the belief that something was wrong, and that with all of my efforts, I shouldn't be having a dry spell. I saw how I was playing out the strategy of trying harder, believing that I could control my states of mind through forced efforts.

What became clear was that absolutely nothing was wrong with how I felt. Experiencing a dry spell is simply one of the many bumps on the spiritual path, and the only problem with it is the one we add, which is to judge it as bad. The strategy of trying harder doesn't allow us to lighten up and just let our experience be as it is, because, to the little mind, this equates with failure. After all, avoiding the feeling of not measuring up is exactly what the strategy of trying harder is designed to do.

Seeing this strategy clearly, and then refraining from our habitual efforts to fix the situation, allows us to simply be with what is. For example, I began to observe my dry spell with a lighthearted curiosity, no longer judging it as bad. And although it didn't immediately disappear, the gloominess surrounding it evaporated, and it was no longer a problem.

If our strategy of control is to try harder, our practice is to bring precision to our observations so we can see our patterns more objectively. We don't need to try to fix ourselves; all we need to do is notice what we do, and then feel the anxiety and contraction in the body that comes from trying to maintain this strategy. Over time, and with perseverance, as we begin to gradually experience the fear underlying this strategy, the controlling behaviors will naturally become less compulsive, and the need to prove ourselves will be held much more lightly.

Seeking Approval

Seeking approval is the second almost universal control strategy. Wanting approval is natural—it's the instinctual survival mode of wanting to be liked in order to fit into the herd. But at a very early age we turn it into something else when we start using approval seeking as a control strategy to mask our insecurities, to avoid feeling the pain of the core delusions of unworthiness. The belief is, "If I can get you to like me, I won't have to feel the pain of being unworthy."

It's amazing how pervasive approval seeking is; in fact, it's almost our default setting as human beings. Since this dynamic is a constant drain on our energy—the energy that we could otherwise use to wake up—we need to bring attention to it in the Me Phase of practice, or else this strategy will succeed at what it does best, blocking our ability to live from our natural Being Kindness.

The need for acceptance often manifests as a pervasive self-consciousness, sometimes accompanied by an anxious quiver in our being, or a subtle tension throughout the body. One student told me that while ordering a cup of coffee, he noticed

he was constantly checking himself to see if he looked accept-
able giving his order, and how he looked standing and waiting,
and how he looked taking the cup in his hand. This may sound
absurd, but as we become more aware, we see how pervasive
self-consciousness can be in ourselves.

Another student said that when she stopped at a red light,
she looked at the car beside her and then in the rearview mirror,
wondering if she looked all right the way she was sitting in her
car. This may sound crazy, or like a trivial thing we shouldn't
waste our time on in spiritual practice, but it is more the norm
than the exception. In order to work with the places where we
are most stuck, we have to acknowledge in ourselves, down to
the last absurd detail, the extent to which we are caught in seeking approval. We can watch ourselves take even a crumb of praise
and turn it into a full-course meal.

We often keep a running dialogue in our minds, possibly to
no one in particular, about how we're doing. Sometimes we feel
the anxiety of not measuring up; other times we feel the inflated
pleasure of doing well. But both the anxiety and the pleasure
come from the same root of needing external confirmation to
feel okay about ourselves. We don't realize that even though it
may feel good when people give us approval, it's really like putting a Band-Aid over a deep wound.

The need for approval may also arise to avoid feeling the anxiety of being separate—the sense of existential disconnect. For
example, if we think we said the wrong thing, we will often
scramble to find ground, to avoid the panic and feelings of being
overwhelmed that come with our potential loss of connection.
Instead of scrambling to find ground, some get paralyzed and
retreat into a protective shell. We're so afraid we can't meet others' standards that we give up. But either strategy—of scrambling to make things right or retreating to avoid failure—keeps
us locked in a cocoon of fear.

47

We may know in our mind that seeking approval is a dead end, and that we can only do so much to please people, but our body still carries the tension of believing that we should be able to please everyone all the time. Of course all of this is based on the core fears of feeling unworthy or of not being enough.

What is the practice here? First we need to notice, notice, notice. Most of the time, we're so caught up in daily life that we don't take time to stop and truly notice all the ways we get caught in trying to please others. However, noticing *without* self-judgment is what allows us to become less identified with our behaviors, and although the need for approval may remain, we will find that it doesn't have to dictate how we live.

Noticing, which doesn't mean self-consciousness, brings self-awareness, and the more we notice, the more subtle that awareness becomes. At some point, we may begin to feel remorse for living from the artificiality of seeking approval. For example, if I become aware of saying things just to get someone to like me, an inner switch starts to come on that tells me I'm disconnecting from myself. This is not the same as guilt, but rather an emotional understanding that we're going against our true nature. Over time, it is this level of understanding that allows our behavior to change on its own.

One other key practice in working with the control strategy of seeking approval is to become able to welcome and say yes to the base fear of unworthiness. Saying yes means we are willing to reside in it—to *feel* it, experiencing it on a visceral level in the body. This may not be easy or comfortable, but it's ultimately much less painful than living in a state of constant anxiety that demands external approval in order to feel OK.

Ultimately, however, we need to know who we are in the larger sense. This means we no longer identify with how others see us, nor do we look to externals to measure our worth; it means instead that we are able to connect with a larger sense of what we're doing on this earth. For example, if I lose touch with a sense of my basic connectedness, or with my primary intention, which is to learn to live from Being Kindness, I can still get caught up in wanting to be admired, or in not wanting to be rejected. But when I connect with a larger sense of what life is, the need for external approval no longer dictates how I feel and live.

We think that we need approval. We think that we need to be loved. But as usual, we have it backward. As we mature spiritually, we discover that we don't *need* to be loved—the real need, if you want to call it that, is *to love*. To love, or to live from Being Kindness, means that we're living from our natural being—from the Zen Heart. But to learn to live from our natural kindness, we usually have to work with what gets in the way, which, in large part, is our deep-seated and pervasive need for approval.

Escaping/Numbing

The third almost universal strategy of control is escaping or numbing, when we either use diversions to escape feeling distressed, or shut off and go numb. Sometimes we go numb on an external level, pretending that an obvious problem doesn't exist. But ignoring the elephant in the room doesn't make it go away, regardless of how much we would like it to disappear. More often we go numb internally, suppressing our unpleasant feelings.

For example, if we lose someone close to us, we will naturally feel sadness and grief. However, it is often difficult to stay with the discomfort of grief, and it is very common to bury the feelings. The practice alternative is to willingly open to the experience. The way we can do this is by breathing the sensations and feelings of sadness and loss into the center of the chest on the in-breath, and then simply breathing out on the out-breath, letting the experience just be. This technique, of breathing into the chest

49

center, will be revisited throughout this book, and its importance can't be overemphasized. It allows us to experience our emotions without getting caught in the drama of Me-stuff. For example, in breathing the sensations of grief—the heaviness, the aching, the longing—into the center of the chest, the sadness may remain, but the melodrama will most likely be gone. Experiencing our feelings in this way, instead of going numb or suppressing them, allows us to live our life in a more open and genuine way.

One other subtle form of numbing is maintaining the belief that we have endless time. This illusion, which to some degree we all hold on to, leaves us convinced that our life will continue indefinitely into the vague future. We are rarely aware of the extent to which this belief has us skating on thin ice, oblivious to the very real fact that our lives can end or be drastically altered at any time, without any warning or preparation. We choose to stay oblivious, to cruise through life on a numbing automatic pilot, so that we don't have to consider anything unpleasant. I'm not saying we should focus on the possibility of bad things happening to us; that would also be a detour from the present reality of our lives. The point is, when we choose a strategy that leaves us living our lives with blinders on, we are not living honestly, nor are we likely to face the things that ultimately need addressing in order to enter into a deeper experience of living.

Much more common than suppressing or going numb is the strategy of seeking diversions, whether it be through entertainment, food, alcohol, drugs, or even staying busy. These addictive behaviors all have one thing in common: avoidance of the pervasive inner feeling of unease. But the relief we get from pursuing this strategy is always temporary, and as we continue to follow these compulsions, we squander energy while still not finding any abiding satisfaction. In fact, our addictive behaviors, whatever they might be, often bring self-judgment and shame, which deplete our energy even further.

Our capacity to understand that life itself doesn't have an agenda, particularly our agenda, seems to be very limited. We insist on our sense of entitlement that life give us comfort, pleasure, and ease. Why can't we understand that the fullest and richest experience of life is often the result of the difficulties that life presents, where we are forced to go deeper? Isn't disappointment often our greatest teacher? To work effectively with our attempts to find comfort through escaping and numbing, it is essential that we first acknowledge this dynamic for what it is—a conditioned control strategy that, again and again, leads only to futility in trying to avoid the inner unease our behaviors are meant to cover over. We should never underestimate our desire to be comfortable; we need to recognize the strength of our desire to avoid both physical and emotional pain.

Two of the more subtle versions of this can be seen in the false comfort we get through pursuing the strategies of self-pity and confusion. Both of these control strategies are very seductive, and both are attempts to avoid feeling our core fears, such as the fear of not being enough in some way or the fear of being wrong. Staying stuck in self-pity or confusion may not seem to have obvious rewards, but we have to understand that we choose to stay stuck in these ways in order to escape the more intense discomfort of our fears.

Once our particular dynamic of escape becomes clear, we have to take the difficult step of refraining from our addictive behaviors. This is very tricky, especially when working with behaviors such as drinking or overeating. Though we may be disciplined enough to stop our addictive behaviors, we may end up doing this merely as behavior modification, without addressing the underlying unease. What is most important in working with our attempts to escape is the willingness to go to the root—to bring awareness to the quiver of unease that we normally don't want to feel. With time, we can do this softly, without gritting our teeth and simply bearing it. With time, we can bring Being Kindness to our efforts, which puts a lot of space around what was once an extremely difficult and seemingly impossible place to be.

For example, if we tend to escape by going to the refrigerator when we feel uneasy, the practice is not to try to eliminate this behavior overnight. Instead, we might simply stand at the refrigerator and for the duration of three breaths, try to fully feel the unease we're trying to cover. Then, we can choose to either eat or refrain from eating. But whatever the outcome, at least we addressed the root of the problem with a little friendliness and lightness, rather than the normal heaviness of our judgmental mind.

It should be obvious at this point that much of the work done in dealing with our various strategies of control, and in fact, much of the work done in the Me Phase of practice, requires understanding our own personal psychology. This is necessary because many of the barriers to living from the spaciousness of Being Awareness or the heart quality of Being Kindness are rooted in our psychological conditioning. We have to see through these barriers—our self-images, our fears, our neediness—in order to connect with awareness of our true nature.

However, the point of working with our emotions and strategies of behavior isn't to become better adjusted, which is closer to the domain of traditional psychology, but to *see and experience* all of the workings of the little self. As we bring experiential awareness to our Me-stuff, the sense of "me" as a separate self slowly begins to dismantle on its own. The more we willingly reside in the unease and separation, the more we see its insubstantiality. This is how we can directly connect with who we truly are and with what our life really is.

4
The Pillars of Practice

AT SOME POINT, everyone on the spiritual path needs to start examining their most basic assumptions, raising questions such as, "What am I doing here?" and "What is the purpose of human life?" If these are just questions of the mind, they can be answered in any number of ways to give us relief. But this relief, which comes from the false sense of control we get primarily through intellectual understanding, will only be temporary. The practice of awakening can never be reduced to an intellectual viewpoint that we then call "truth." To avoid falling into the trap of accepting conceptual explanations, we need to focus, *experientially*, on the essential human problem that practice addresses: that we don't know who we are, that we feel disconnected from our true nature.

Does this mean that we shouldn't talk about practice? No—it just means that we should be aware that we need to be clear what it is that we're talking about. In fact, our actual practice is quite straightforward, having three distinct and very specific pillars: daily sitting, practicing with everyday life, and deepening practice through meditation retreats.

Daily Meditation

The first pillar is the still, silent sitting of meditation, where the body and mind can gradually settle down. Here's a good analogy:

Picture a glass full of clear water with a layer of mud at the bottom. Now imagine stirring the water—what remains is swirling muddy water. This swirling muddy water is the life of Me-stuff—full of anxiety and confusion. We live our lives trying to maintain control, but with little clarity about what we're doing. The result: we'll continue to race around with little direction.

When we take the glass and set it down, the mud begins to settle to the bottom, and what we're left with is a glass of clear, still water. Likewise, when we sit down to meditate, our spinning mind will gradually slow down, and the normal low-key agitation in the body will feel more settled. This settling is not just a psychological phenomenon; it happens in the physical body as well. There is something very settling about not moving when the energy of agitation goes through us. As we learn to stay still, we no longer feed the agitation, we no longer stir up the water.

However, often it's extremely difficult to stay still; and it is true that equanimity does not always occur. Sometimes the spinning mind will continue to spin despite our best efforts to stay still. In fact, sometimes, even in the midst of stillness, some deeply held agitation will rise to the surface of awareness. Nonetheless, over time, still, silent sitting generates a settled quality, one we can tap into even in the middle of the muddy turmoil of everyday life.

Along with staying still, another important factor in sitting is our posture. Many teachers emphasize the need to sit in an erect posture, in part to help keep the mind alert. While sitting erect is generally recommended, I don't believe the physical posture we take is nearly as important as the mental posture. The sense of intention and presence, which is crucial to sitting, is certainly not dependent on a particular physical posture. For example, when I had a long period of illness, I had to meditate lying down because I didn't have the strength to sit cross-legged. At first I thought I wouldn't be able to truly meditate while lying down, but it gradually became clear to me that as long as my intention was strong, the physical posture was not so important. Still, as comfort-seeking humans, we always have to be careful that our need for comfort doesn't undermine our sitting. One reason to stay still and to maintain a disciplined posture is to keep our craving for comfort from determining how we sit. Never underestimate the sense of entitlement to comfort.

There is an appendix at the end of this book that gives basic meditation instructions, but it is certainly worthwhile to find a good meditation teacher who can give you instructions in person. If nothing else, this may help you find a posture that suits your physical situation while still allowing you to maintain a sense of discipline. Having ongoing contact with a meditation teacher can also help with both initial technique and the many difficulties that are bound to arise in our ongoing effort to awaken. The little mind is very tricky, presenting numerous roadblocks and detours that take us off the path. For example, one thing to always watch for is the tendency to push too hard, trying to get somewhere. While discipline and effort are undoubtedly important, strain is not. We can be serious about practice without being somber and grim.

Along with developing a good posture, we also need to learn what to do with the mind. I usually suggest that students start periods of meditation with a focused attention on the breath, in order to bypass the busy mind. This makes it easier for the mind and body to settle down. The instruction is to actually feel the specific sensations of the breath, such as the coolness in the nostrils on the in-breath, and the feelings of expansion and contraction in the chest and belly as we inhale and exhale. If the mind is particularly busy, as will often happen, the added instruction is to count the breath from one to ten, counting on the exhalation only. You would begin again at one each time you got to ten, or each time you found yourself caught in a thought loop. As the mind settles, awareness expands beyond just the breath to include other sensations in the body, as well as environmental input, such as sounds or air temperature. The practice is just to be awake and aware. Please note that this simple-sounding instruction can be very difficult to do.

Part of the learning process in meditation is becoming aware of any beliefs we have about what meditation should look like. Perhaps one of the biggest roadblocks is the deep-seated assumption that meditation will make us feel better. But meditation is not necessarily about feeling calm or clear or relaxed. These states will certainly occur, yet we are missing the point if we focus on having pleasant or special experiences. Meditation is about being awake—to *whatever* we feel. It is about simply being here, including experiencing the states and feelings that we don't like. So one of the major aspects of a meditation practice is to learn to attend to whatever arises in the mind, whether we like it or not. Trying to achieve a particular state of mind keeps us stuck in the self-centered world of Me-stuff. In fact, grasping after a particular state of mind only perpetuates the grasping mind—the I-as-a-me. By contrast, paying objective awareness to the small self allows us, paradoxically, to connect with the larger self of Being Awareness.

One thing we have to pay a great deal of attention to is the attachment to our thoughts. The specific practice of thought labeling is perhaps the most helpful tool in learning to observe our thoughts with clarity. This in turn allows us to see the depth of our attachment to our thinking; and until we work in this area, we will be at the mercy of our conditioned beliefs. Thought labeling entails silently repeating a thought verbatim. For example, during meditation, if we notice ourselves entertaining the thought "Sitting is too hard," we label it by saying, "Having a believed thought: 'sitting is too hard.'" This process helps us break our identification with a particular thought, in a sense removing our investment or belief in it. One of the crucial insights in practice is when we learn to see our thoughts merely as thoughts, and not as The Truth.

Naturally, we don't specifically label every thought; if we did, sitting would be much too busy. Most thoughts can be labeled generically, in categories such as "planning," "conversing," "fantasizing," and so on. Once we notice our own particular pattern of thinking, we simply say the one word that best fits our pattern rather than labeling the entire believed thought. However, with thoughts that carry a heavy emotional load, it's still useful to label them specifically, because these are the thoughts that are most likely to determine how we feel and act.

Seeing clearly what the mind believes is an essential aspect of sitting; another is staying present with the physical experience in the body. This is very difficult to do, both because it is often uncomfortable and because we have very little training in this area. The one tool that I've found most helpful in staying with our present-moment experience is using the koan-question "What is this?" This question is followed by coming back again and again to the physical reality of our body and the environment. The answer to this question is never what our experience is "about," which is a mental concern, but instead points to the actual visceral or felt experience in the moment.

Using this lifetime koan regularly brings a sense of curiosity to our sitting—simply wanting to know the truth of the moment. This kind of curiosity takes us out of the self-centered orientation of the Me Phase of practice and into the more spacious perspective of Being Awareness. The less we are *caught* in the clouds of our thoughts and emotions, the more we can *relate to* them from the sky quality of awareness. And as we cultivate a curiosity that's willing to look at whatever arises, we also tap into the quality of Being Kindness, in that we are no longer judging our experience, or ourselves, as bad; instead, we welcome it nonjudgmentally.

Learning to approach our sitting with the curiosity and friendliness of "What is this?" mind will gradually extend into our everyday life. In fact, if our sitting doesn't eventually impact our daily living—for example, if we can sit in calmness and spaciousness but still react emotionally in the same way as always in our daily life—then our practice is missing the point. Sitting is the pillar that allows us to cultivate the qualities of perseverance, curiosity, presence, and Being Kindness, but we still have to work at bringing these qualities into everyday living.

Daily Life: Difficulties and Mindfulness

The second pillar of practice is working with everyday life, including difficulties that range from being cut off on the freeway to issues concerning relationships, money, and work. Regardless of how subtle or extreme the difficulty is, the practice is the same—learning how to use these very difficulties to become increasingly free from conditioning and the constriction of fear.

In the last twenty years, this aspect of practice has been given increasing attention, but more often than not, the attention doesn't go much beyond the injunction to make everyday life a part of practice. Often, there are few instructions on the specifics of how to do this. And since our conditioning runs very deep, without specific instructions we're likely to revert to addressing our difficulties through trying to achieve a state of calm or spaciousness. But until we make the difficult efforts to free ourselves from the deeply ingrained programming from our early years, these patterns will continue to play out in our daily living.

The first step in working with difficulties in everyday life is developing the understanding that our difficulties are, in fact, an important part in our path of awakening. We often forget that disappointment can be our best teacher. We forget that adversity is necessary on the spiritual path, and that it's actually our good fortune that life's hardships will often push us in ways that we would rarely push ourselves on our own. Without the difficulties of everyday life, and a practice approach that prepares us to be present to them, it is unlikely that our practice would ever penetrate though the layers of armoring and conditioning that are firmly in place.

Once we have this understanding—that practice includes *everything*—we can begin to use the specific tools that are learned in the first pillar of silent sitting. For example, when caught in emotional distress, it's always crucial to clearly see our thoughts, our requirements, our expectations. And it's equally important that we ask with a curious mind, "What is this?" And then rest in the answer, which is always our physical experience in the moment.

Both of these practice tools—seeing our thoughts clearly and physically feeling the reality of our life—are enhanced as we cultivate the mind-set that's willing to welcome a difficulty, to say yes to it. This mind-set grows with the increasing unwillingness to stay complacent. Saying yes allows us to move toward unknown territory, even while the voice of fear tells us to stop. As we understand that without this step we will forever remain stuck, there's a willingness to enter into life in a new way.

Practicing with our daily life on this level is particularly difficult when the mind is reeling in self-doubt and confusion. At such times, how do we return to the heart that seeks to awaken? When everything seems dark and unworkable, when our aspiration has grown dim, one thing we can always do is take a deep breath into the center of the chest, and on the out-breath extend to ourselves the same warmth and compassion we would extend to a loved one in duress. Breathing into the heart, physically connecting with the center of our being, extends Being Kindness to ourselves even when there appears to be no Being Kindness in sight. This helps break though the layers of armoring and protection that we've all erected in the false hope that it will make us feel more secure. At first, we may only be capable of doing this for one or two breaths at a time. But we have to realize, especially when caught in despair, that our conditioning goes very deep, and truly freeing ourselves from these embedded emotional reactions can take a long time. Understanding this, we're less likely to be hard on ourselves. And very slowly, as we hold on to our pretenses and self-images less tightly, it becomes possible to extend Being Kindness inward for longer and longer periods of time, thereby reconnecting with a more heartfelt sense of what life is.

In a way, our efforts to become more awake in everyday life are analogous to how we nourish the body by choosing to eat a healthy diet. Instead of repeating our conditioned behaviors that feed the growth of the little self—the I-as-a-me—we bring awareness to them, seeing what beliefs are at work, and willingly residing in the accompanying physical experience. Every moment of trying to be more awake feeds I-as-Awareness, enabling our experience of life to move beyond the confines of the narrow world of I-as-a-me to the more spacious sense of Being Awareness.

Working with our everyday life difficulties is not the only way to cultivate Being Awareness. There is also an emphasis on living more awake, which means being more tuned in to our senses, to people, to the environment. The emphasis is on being here, not just on working with problems. Living more awake often includes specific techniques that foster the nonconceptual experiencing of reality, beyond the thought world where we normally spend so much time. One such daily-life practice that many students have found helpful is using "daily menu" items, where each day you focus on a different area of practice. For example, one day it might be listening to sounds attentively, starting from the moment you wake up and continuing until you go to sleep. Over time, this develops the ability to hear not only the obvious external sounds but the very subtle ones as well. Furthermore, you learn to listen with your whole body, not just with your ears. Other examples of "menu" practices include staying with the breath as it enters and exits the chest center, observing shadows, being very aware of your hands, and on and on.

Menu practices help get us out of our heads and into a more physical experience of reality. We might take a short aphorism as our menu item for the day, returning to the phrase over and over again as an anchor to what's important. For example, one of my favorites is hearing the Zen bird on my shoulder asking, "Is today the day you're going to die?" I don't think of this as a somber reflection, but rather as a reminder to lightly reflect on what is most important. Other phrases I find useful are "Just this" or "What is practice in this moment?" or "What am I experiencing right now?" There is a list of additional practice reminders in the appendix called "The Essential Reminders."

One other particularly good menu practice using a phrase is to substitute the word it for the word I. So instead of saying, "I'm anxious," or "I'm hurt," we would say, "It's anxious," or "It's hurt." By saying "it," our identification with our emotion—with I-as-a-me—is undermined. The less we identify with I-as-a-me, the less we will require approval and the less we will fear being hurt. As we no longer carry the emotional-bodily tension that accompanies our me-centered preoccupation, we can increasingly live with a sense of ease and equanimity.

In working with menu practices, you can use whatever phrases or tools are most relevant to you, as long as they serve the purpose of getting you out of the narrow mental world of Me-stuff and into a more spacious sense of what life is. Every time we remember the phrase, or remember the more sensory-based menu practices, such as listening to sounds, we are feeding I-as-Awareness.

This kind of intention and focused effort invites a larger experience of what life is, using everyday life as one of the main pillars of our practice.

Retreats

The third pillar of practice is the emphasis on regularly attending meditation retreats, where we have the opportunity to settle into all aspects of practice more deeply. Retreats create an artificial environment, minimizing external distractions so that we can look more deeply inward. Meditation retreats usually last from three to ten days. Often they begin at five or six in the morning and don't end until nine or ten at night. Retreats may vary greatly from place to place: some are done in complete silence, while others allow some talking. Many retreats stress strict adherence to procedures and rituals, but there are also retreats that are much more casual. Most often meditation retreats involve many periods of sitting and walking meditation. At Zen Center San Diego, where we stress both silence and still sitting, we recommend that students start with shorter retreats so that they don't feel overwhelmed. We also include frequent consultations with the teachers, to allow students the opportunity to clarify the many questions and issues that may arise during a retreat.

Since participants may feel both the physical discomfort from long days of sitting and the emotional discomfort that comes as our Pandora's box of emotions slowly opens, retreats can be, in part, an act of "conscious suffering," where we intentionally place ourselves in circumstances where we are forced to deal with difficulty. The retreat environment can push us in ways that we would never push ourselves on our own. But in doing this intentionally, with the idea of using our suffering to become more awake, we are cultivating I-as-Awareness. Every time we make an effort to stay with our experience, especially when it's difficult, it is food for our being, nourishing qualities like perseverance and equanimity. And because retreats offer us the opportunity to make these efforts throughout the day, day after day, they become one of the prime ways our learning can go deeper.

Students often judge retreats as good or bad depending on how they feel when it's over. If they feel calm and spacious, it's thought of as a good retreat. If they feel discouraged or confused, it's usually considered a bad retreat. But the real criterion for the quality of a retreat is not how we feel but what we have learned, which can be very subtle, and perhaps not obvious right away. Sometimes we may feel very low at the end of a retreat and not even know what we learned until days after the retreat is over. I remember once being very discouraged when a retreat ended, even questioning why I had made the effort to come. But several hours later, as I was sitting on a plane going back home, the veil between me and "reality" rose on its own, bringing a clarity that was deeper than anything I had ever experienced before. I wasn't doing anything on the plane to make this happen; but what I had judged as wasted efforts at the retreat just needed time to be assimilated. After that experience, I began to look at retreats very differently, no longer judging them based on how I felt, but rather seeing them as opportunities to learn on a deeper level.

When I talk about learning, I'm not talking about acquiring conceptual knowledge, where we accumulate more facts; in practice, the learning process is experiential. Without the experiential component, without our inner struggles, our understanding remains merely conceptual. For practice to be transformative, we must move from growth in mere knowledge to growth in Being Awareness. This does not mean, however, that there is a bigger or better "me"; what it means is that we are connecting more fully with who we really are and with what life is.

As an example of the learning process in retreats, a very common meditation instruction is to bring attention to the breath.

At first, we usually understand this to mean we should focus on the breath in a very concentrated way. So when we go to retreats, we will follow this practice, often with the idea that if we stay really focused on the breath, we will become calm. This notion is what most people believe meditation is about in the Me Phase of practice.

After we've worked with this practice for a while, our understanding may begin to change. As we sit and struggle through the long hours of retreats, there is often a shift from simply trying to become calm toward viewing the breath as part of a wider container of awareness—the space within which we experience our thoughts and emotions. At this point we are moving from the Me Phase of practice into Being Awareness, cultivating a larger sense of life.

But the awareness of the breath can take us even deeper over time. As we practice awareness of the breath through many retreats, it can become a touch point or portal into reality. Eventually, a very light, almost effortless awareness replaces the former disciplined focus on the breath. At some point we become aware of the breath breathing itself, like a breeze that goes right through us, without real effort. The breath touches lightly on the heart, and puts us in touch naturally with the warmth of Being Kindness. Paradoxically, this is both wonderful and also nothing special.

In short, using the breath for awareness can be understood very differently; but to go beyond the mental realm, our understanding must be grounded in our inner struggle to awaken. This is but one of the many ways that retreats are so valuable, offering us the opportunity to take our learning to deeper levels, always grounded in our own experience.

These are three of the main pillars of spiritual practice—sitting still in meditation, working with everyday life, and attending retreats. But please remember, we still have to come back again and again to the bigger picture of practice, which is to become awake to what life really is, and to live from the Being Kindness that is our true nature.

Unless these pillars of practice are seen within this greater context, it's very easy to get caught in a more myopic view of practice—seeing practice as just about still sitting, or just about clarifying our psychological conditioning, or just about the deeper learning that is possible at retreats. Practice is not just about anything. The more inclusive view includes all of the pillars, and yet it is in no way limited or defined by them.

5

Three Breaths Practice

SOMETIMES THE SIMPLEST practice techniques are also the ones that are most effective. Granted, all techniques can be misused; we can easily turn them into instruments for self-improvement rather than using them as tools to wake up. We can also get lost in the techniques themselves and forget about the bigger picture of practice. Nonetheless, focusing on techniques may be essential for a very long time. Then, gradually, all good techniques tend to dismantle themselves as the inherent teaching becomes a part of who we are.

The Conscious Pause

One simple but very effective technique is called the Three Breaths Practice. Normally, there are many times throughout the day when we "come to"—that is, when we simply become aware. Unfortunately, most of the time, these moments last only a few seconds; afterward, we fall right back into waking sleep, where we are basically unaware, lost in our thoughts or in our personal drama. Observation of your own process will verify that this is true. The Three Breaths Practice is a way of helping to extend these moments of awareness, not just during sitting but throughout our day-to-day living.

The Three Breaths Practice involves injecting a conscious pause in the middle of our usual state of waking sleep, a pause that lasts for the duration of three full breaths. Here's how it works: whenever you "come to" for a moment, you make the conscious intention to stay there for at least three full breaths. You don't necessarily focus just on the breath itself, but bring awareness to your entire experience in that moment, whatever it may be.

For example, if you "wake up" in the midst of impatience, you don't try to become patient. You simply feel—fully feel— the visceral texture of the present-moment experience, impatience and all. The commitment is to reside in the experience for the duration of three full breaths.

There's a very definite sensation of "being here" that can be cultivated by the Three Breaths Practice. Try this brief experiment: First, bring attention to your breath, feeling the coolness as it enters the nostrils. Staying with the sensations of the breath, also experience the room. And staying with the air and the room, now bring awareness to the overall experience of the body. Don't focus on specific sensations but instead on the overall feeling, or gestalt, of the body in space, the sense of your own presence, or being, just sitting there, breathing and being in the room. Now stay with this, with as much of your attention as you can bring, for three full breaths. If you can do this, you'll recognize the experience as one of being present, of being here, in the sense of expanding beyond your customary limiting perceptual boundaries.

One of the reasons the Three Breaths Practice is so helpful is that it's something you can actually do without a strong or prolonged effort. It's brief and simple, and you can do it many times throughout the day, regardless of how you are feeling. In fact, it might be just as beneficial to try this practice when you are feeling happy and carefree as it is to try it when you are feeling emotionally low.

We all know that it's not enough to simply want to wake up;

the forces of sleep are powerful and unrelenting. Yet, this one simple practice, which is often not particularly difficult, can begin to bring moments of clarity and presence to our normal fog of waking sleep. Just settle into the moment and remind yourself to "feel this"—for at least three full breaths.

Staying with Distress

Another interesting and very effective use of the Three Breaths Practice is when we find ourselves in the midst of a painful or distressing experience. Usually it is very difficult to stay focused at such times, since we have a natural aversion to discomfort. But by using the Three Breaths Practice, it's often possible to "make a deal" with the resisting ego by telling it that you will only stay with the discomfort for the duration of three breaths.

The ego is willing to make this arrangement because it maintains the illusion of control—which is the main goal of the ego. So the practice is to tell your small mind that you will only feel the distress for three full breaths, after which it can decide what to focus on. Be sure not to renege on the deal; after the three breaths you allow yourself to drift into your normal diversions. Then, after a time, you make the same arrangement, feeling the distress again, for three breaths at a time.

What's amazing about this particular nuance of the Three Breaths Practice is that the ego is so willing to go along. Often the resistance we feel makes our difficult experiences that much more difficult. But when the resistance is abated, even if only for three breaths at a time, it becomes clear that what we are resisting is only deeply believed thoughts and sometimes intense physical sensations. The more often we enter into and feel these moments of discomfort, the more we understand that it's more painful to push away the experience than it is to actually feel it. We learn this pivotal understanding three breaths at a time.

Addictive Tendencies

One last use of the Three Breaths Practice is when we are caught in one of our addictive tendencies, such as fantasizing, surfing the Web, or staying very busy. These tendencies are often seductive, and we normally have very little interest in giving them up. But as in staying with distress, it's possible to make a deal with the ego—in this case in the ego's guise of the addictive mind—by making the arrangement to come back to reality for just three breaths, after which you will willingly go back into your habitual behavior.

For example, say you're sitting at your computer, mindlessly going from one thing to another, just filling up time with addictive busyness. Perhaps you "wake up" for a moment and become aware of what you're doing. It would be unrealistic to think that you could then just stop and get up—we all know that addictions are not very amenable to reason or even self-discipline. But the one thing the addictive mind might be willing to do is take a three-breath pause, mainly because it knows it will take over the wheel again very soon.

For the duration of three full breaths, we fully feel the experience of addiction. This is a physical experience, and includes the sense of speed and energy in the body. You're not trying to break the addiction, but rather to feel the discomfort that drives the addictive behavior. After the three breaths, you let yourself go back to waking sleep. Then, after a time you make the arrangement again. And then again. What you may find is that after doing this several times, the circuitry of the seductive power of the addiction is naturally broken.

The only way to experience the value of the Three Breaths Practice is to try it. All that is required is to bring a conscious intention to your practice for three breaths at a time. This is admittedly a very simple technique, but it's important to do what we can, when we can, and gradually the small efforts accumulate and begin to impact the quality of our lives. Practice is not an all-or-nothing endeavor.

PART TWO

The Foundations of Being Awareness

6

Qualities of Awakening

WHAT PRACTICES are most effective in helping us awaken? What are the most essential qualities that we need to bring to practice? Three qualities that I have found to be absolutely essential on the path to an awakened life are perseverance, curiosity, and mercy. Without these it would be very difficult to move from the Me Phase to the phases of Being Awareness or Being Kindness.

Perseverance

As you may know, ups and downs in practice are predictable and inevitable. In fact, one sign of a maturing practice is remembering to anticipate the downs, to anticipate resistance, and to know what practice entails at those times. For example, when we've been to enough meditation retreats, we know that if we have a particularly strong retreat, sometime after the retreat ends we're likely to be hit with an equal wave of resistance. It may not happen right away, but it will likely happen sooner or later. What is the countermeasure when resistance arises? Isn't it always to persevere?

Perseverance means that we are steadfast, regardless of how we feel. Even when we don't feel motivated, or can't quite remember why we're practicing, at least we know the necessity of not giving up. We know the need to at least show up. In fact, persevering, in the face of discouragement and resistance, is often where our learning goes deepest. There are times for all of us when resistance can be very powerful, where we may feel totally lost in our quest. Who hasn't experienced thoughts such as "I'll never get this," "I'll never make the efforts that are necessary," or "What's the point?" Yet, to continue to practice—to persevere—even when we don't remember why, is how we learn to go deeper into our life. Just staying with the visceral or physical experience of doubt—the knowing that we don't know—is how we enter most deeply into practice.

At one point, when I was very involved at a Zen center in Northern California, I was hit, seemingly out of the blue, with a wall of resistance, and I didn't want to sit anymore, nor did I want to go to the center. But even though I couldn't stand being there, something in me knew not to bolt. I forced myself to go to just one sitting a week, basically hanging on by a thread. Then, after a few months, the resistance began to fade, and I reentered the practice with a deeper involvement than before, not only internally but also in the external activities at the center. The point is, sometimes simply persevering will allow us to move through even the worst resistance. Even when our practice efforts seem to produce very little in terms of tangible results, with the little mind seeing "failure" at every step, a part of us knows that we have no choice but to keep starting over. This is the only way we will ever go deeper into our life.

Perseverance, on the most basic practical level, might mean that we meditate every day, regardless of whether or not we feel like it. It might also mean that we show up regularly at a practice center, and attend retreats, even though often we'd rather be somewhere else. Perseverance also means that we stay present with our most difficult experiences, even if it's just for three breaths at a time, and even when a part of us wants to escape into thinking, fantasizing, judging, or blaming—whatever our favorite detour is.

Perseverance requires a kind of courage, the courage to look deeply into our beliefs, and particularly to uncover our illusions about ourselves. It also takes courage to examine what we are doing with our lives—to look at ourselves with unflinching honesty and say, "Yes, I do that" or "Yes, I get stuck there." This is not the same as self-judgment; it's simply objective self-observation. Yet, from that deep looking, we gradually develop the sense of purpose that makes practice the central orientation of our life. The quest to know what life really is, and to live open-heartedly, becomes our main focus, and also the context within which everything else is seen, making it possible to welcome our life regardless of circumstances.

During this process, there is a point at which an essential shift occurs in our being, where we move from a predominant orientation toward sleep and mechanicalness—whose primary goals are comfort, security, approval, and control—to a growing orientation toward wanting to live more awake. This shift is not like a change in mood, or a temporary phase, or even a change in attitude; it is an actual change in our way of being. This shift deepens our willingness to persevere, and although strong emotions and old patterns may resurface once in a while, fundamentally there is no turning back from practice. Without this shift in our being we will always be at the mercy of our moods, desires, opinions, and emotions, as well as of our ever-changing external circumstances. In other words, we will perpetuate our old ways of seeing and being, thereby maintaining a life of sleep and mechanicalness.

So what is it that changes? And how? First we have to ask, who are we to begin with? For example, what is an "Ezra" other than a physical body with a personality? Yet, don't we try to protect this "me" at all costs? To make the change or transformation that's possible through practice, we first have to see how serious we are about the little things—our upsets, our discomforts, and so on, without being serious enough about the bigger things, such as realizing our true nature. We're uncomfortable when we feel rejected, lonely, or unappreciated, but we're not nearly uncomfortable enough about how asleep we are, or how self-centered we are. Nor do we often enough feel the discomfort of how disconnected we are from ourselves and others, and how rarely we experience the love that is our nature. Remember, I'm not talking about making punitive self-judgments; I'm talking about seeing clearly the nature and magnitude of sleep within ourselves.

One of the first steps in the transformative process of waking up is seeing with precision all of the little "me's" that make up the protective cocoon of our persona. This is the work of the Me Phase of practice. For example, we begin to notice the often unconscious voices that say, I want comfort; I want security; I want approval; I want control; I want to feel worthy; I want to feel loved; and I want not to feel fear, or loneliness, or rejection. These voices bind together to form the seeming solidity of a "me."

In observing these "I's" or "me's" with precision, the "I" that is observing—which could be called our aspiration—begins to grow. When we experience the clash between the I-that-wants (comfort, control, etc.) and what life is actually presenting, the practice is to persevere, to stay with what is. When we do this, the I-that-aspires-to-awaken grows. It is almost as if the physical energy that is generated from our conscious struggles feeds the growth of our aspiration, and transforms into Being Awareness, or I-as-Awareness. Similarly, every time we indulge the I-that-wants, we strengthen the I-as-a-me. In the never-ending struggle between what I want and what is, a real perseverance develops, making it possible to be with what is, regardless of whether or not we like it. Thus, the priority shifts from "what I want" to the aspiration to wake up.

To stay with our experience in this way requires a pivotal understanding: that there is no turning back from practice. In the ongoing struggle, we may begin to see through our so-called needs, our fears, our very solid identities; and slowly, our conscious efforts strengthen I-as-Awareness. Remember, this is not a mental struggle—it is not about thinking differently; rather it comes from getting out of our heads and into our bodies—that is, into the physical experience of the present moment.

When I-as-Awareness grows, everything changes. But for this change to take place, we must persevere in our efforts to turn away from constantly trying to seek comfort and avoid pain. We must experience more and more deeply the objective anguish of living disconnected from ourselves. Only then will we be motivated to rethink our priorities. Only then will we be able to bring a seriousness of purpose to the only thing that warrants such sincerity—the genuine path to reconnecting with the heart. Once we truly enter this path, there is no turning back.

Curiosity—Saying Yes

Though perseverance is essential, it is not enough by itself. With perseverance alone, it is tempting to become almost militant and stoic in practice. We might even become grim. So to balance this essential component, we also have to cultivate the softer quality of curiosity.

Curiosity means that we're willing to explore unknown territory—the places the ego doesn't want to go. Curiosity allows us to take a step at our edge, toward our deepest fears. Unfortunately, our innate curiosity is often stifled at an early age. Our wanting to know, as well as our natural delight in knowing, is easily covered over by seeking approval or predictability, and is therefore hard to access.

Asking the koan-question "What is this?" is the essence of practicing with curiosity, in that the only "answer" comes from being open to actually experiencing the truth of each moment. Being truly curious means we're willing to say yes to our experience, even the hard parts, instead of indulging the no of our habitual resistance.

Saying yes doesn't mean we like our experience, or that we necessarily *feel* accepting. It doesn't even mean that we override the no. Saying yes simply means that we pay attention—meticulous attention—to the no. It means we're no longer resisting the people, things, and fears that we don't like; instead we're learning to open to them in order to experience what's actually going on.

One definition of practice is the willingness to be with our life as it is. But this is a difficult concept to comprehend: that practice is not about having a particular state of mind, such as calmness, or being free from problems. Furthermore, understanding this intellectually is very different from understanding it with the core of our being.

This is not to deny that through practice we will, in fact, experience more equanimity, and that problems will not seem so burdensome. But, ironically, when we demand that life be a particular way it almost guarantees the opposite—a continuing state of unease and dissatisfaction.

Here's something to consider: Can you imagine the possibility of having anxiety and not being anxious about it? Or having depression and not being depressed about it? In other words, can you imagine feeling discomfort without trying to get rid of it? The question is, how do we learn to live in this way? There is no easy answer, but the key is to learn how to welcome—with curiosity—whatever our life is in each moment.

The deeply ingrained human attitude that we need to be free from problems is really one of our greatest problems. For example, when something unpleasant happens, we'll almost always react from the deeply held belief that life *should* be free from discomfort and pain. We might not even be conscious of having this belief, but because we believe it, it colors (or discolors) how we relate to reality.

What happens when we no longer cling to the belief that we have to be free from problems? Pick one small problem that you have (and don't want), and ask yourself what it would be like if you could actually say yes when this problem arose, moving toward it voluntarily, consciously, with curiosity?

This is not a masochistic attitude; rather, it's the actual (and often gentle) willingness to stop pushing our experience away and demanding that life be different. When we learn what it means to say yes to a difficulty, to be curious about what life is, our whole world turns right side up; it allows us to experience life more as an adventure than as a nightmare. This is similar to how we approach meditation retreats, where we come knowing it may be difficult, yet we're willing, at least to some degree, to explore whatever arises.

In my early retreats, I was so intimidated that I often had to stoically grit my teeth to get through them. But later, when I learned to bring curiosity to the adverse reactions that would arise, I'd simply say to myself, "Here it comes again; what will it be like this time?"

Can you see the difference between these two attitudes? The grim stoicism is really another way of saying no, whereas invoking curiosity is the beginning of saying yes. Bringing curiosity allows a kind of spaciousness to envelop even our most difficult experiences. We are no longer so caught up in "me and my difficulty," but more able to relate to the difficulty from a larger sense of what life is. This is the spaciousness of Being Awareness, which lets us feel a sense of equanimity even in the midst of our distress. This equanimity comes from willingly residing in our experience, from opening to it with curiosity.

However, to be honest, most of the time when disruptive experiences arise, we feel jangled, and our unspoken thought is that something is wrong. We might even think that being upset is the only possible response. And further, we will probably believe that something needs to be fixed—that we need to get calm or clear or relaxed.

But try to imagine relating to a difficult experience without seeing it as a problem. For example, if you truly welcomed a distressing event as an opportunity to learn, wouldn't the same event then become nourishment for your being rather than poison for the body? In fact, the distressful event can motivate us to work with *exactly* what we need to work with. Ultimately, practice requires the implicit understanding that whatever situation or emotion we can't say yes to is the exact direction of our path.

I mentioned earlier that it's possible to have anxiety but not *be* anxious about it. Take the simple example of having anxiety around making a phone call where the conversation is likely to be unpleasant. When the anxiety arises, the unspoken thought is usually that something is wrong, and more so, that something is wrong with me or with them. And, of course, we feel that we need to calm down.

However, from a practice point of view, having anxiety doesn't mean that something is bad. All it means is that there is anxiety, which is simply the result of our own particular conditioning. We don't have to fight it. Nor do we need to fix it. In fact, when anxiety predictably arises, instead of viewing it as a problem, we simply pause, acknowledge it, and then say yes to it—which means welcoming it with curiosity as an opportunity to work with our own particular edge.

We don't have to like the anxiety. We just need to feel it as the physical experience that it is. And when we rest in it and learn from it, we no longer identify with the I-as-anxious, but rather with the I-as-Awareness—the spaciousness of Being Awareness. Within that larger sense of being, the anxiety is not a particular problem.

Sometimes it seems that we can't say yes to our experience. Perhaps the experience is too powerful or too overwhelming. Perhaps it feels like death itself. When we find ourselves in the midst of such a painful or distressing experience, usually it is very difficult to stay present with it. This is normal, because we have a natural aversion to discomfort, and as a consequence, our resistance can be very strong.

The voice of fear tells us we have reached an edge beyond which we're unwilling to go. Yet, our curiosity tells us to take one more step forward. Fear says no!—it warns us to close and defend; but another part of us says yes!—calling us to open and connect. Saying yes to life means saying yes to everything, even longing, fear, and pain. The way we do this is by breathing the uncomfortable sensations directly into the center of the chest on the in-breath; then on the out-breath simply breathing out. As we bring the distressing emotions into the center of the chest, we can experience the healing power of the heart. This *nonconceptual* experience allows us to become truly intimate with our life. The fundamental point is that until we become intimate with our fears, until we can welcome them with curiosity, they will always limit our ability to love. In other words, the path to Being Kindness requires giving our willing attention to the very things that seem to block the way.

Mercy

The third quality of awakening, along with perseverance and curiosity, is something that is often overlooked—the quality of mercy. Mercy is sometimes referred to as loving-kindness, but whatever we call it, it is a quality that is necessary throughout the practice life, and it is an essential aspect of the third phase of Being Kindness. The word mercy may turn some people away if they fear a false sentimentality, an airy-fairy approach that is contrary to the rigorous approach they imagine practice must entail. But what we're actually talking about is the ability to abandon the harshness of the judgmental mind. After all, isn't it the judgmental mind that runs the constant subliminal message that we're not good enough, and that we never will be?

Without mercy, we cut ourselves off from the heart, which means we also cut ourselves off from others. Without mercy, our practice will always have that hard edge created by the mind that's constantly judging, evaluating, finding fault. For instance, when breathing into the center of the chest, which is an essential part of the Being Kindness meditations, the mind might say, "Shouldn't you be doing something more tangible and worthwhile?" This is the voice of the ego, not wanting to give up control, not wanting to feel vulnerable. Perhaps there is the underlying belief "I must be hard on myself or else I'll falter." This view is completely upside down, and sadly it leads some people to miss out on the essential quality of mercy, a quality that goes all the way back to the teachings of both Jesus and the Buddha, as well as other spiritual traditions.

It might be worthwhile to look at your views in this area a little more deeply. What strong beliefs arise when you hear the word mercy? What do you really fear when you withhold mercy? What prevents you from applying to yourself the basic tenderness and compassion that you would to a loved one in duress?

Mercilessness is an aspect of the judging mind. Mercy is a quality of the heart—the heart that is spacious beyond the mind's imagination. No matter how serious we are about practice, no matter how much we persevere with techniques, no matter how curious we are, without the quality of mercy we will always stay stuck in the mind's judgment.

Almost every teacher and every book on practice will emphasize the need to be gentle with ourselves. This is not a new message. The problem is how to do it. What does it actually mean to be kind to ourselves? How do we generate kindness when everything in us is feeling just the opposite?

One way of cultivating mercy is by knowing ourselves deeply—seeing through all of our so-called faults, our imagined unworthiness, our deepest fears. The more we come to know these aspects of ourselves, the more we develop a benign tolerance, not only for ourselves but also for the whole human drama. Every time a negative core-belief judgment arises, we have to see it and label it with precision. We have to observe our tendency to judge, over and over, until we learn to see it as nothing but the conditioning that it is. And then we have to stay with the subtle felt sense of contraction in the body— whether it's heaviness, sogginess, feeling crumbled, feeling lost, or whatever. Much of this work is done in the Me Phase of practice.

We are often merciless in our self-judgments—not only when we're upset at ourselves but as an ongoing frame of mind. What is a negative core belief if not an ongoing negative self-judgment about who we are, such as the belief that I'm unworthy? Such judgments are always lurking under the surface, waiting to arise.

Here's a good example: one night when I was scheduled to have personal practice-related consultations with students, I first went up to the meditation room. I often sit with students until the bell rings to officially start the sitting, at which point I leave to conduct the consultations. But on this night, when I went to the meditation room, there was only one student present. My attendant wasn't there, nor was the timekeeper. I thought to myself, "Well, that's okay—what am I, a prima donna? I can ring the bell and announce the consultations myself if necessary." But by the time the meditation session was supposed to start, there was still only one student in the room. So there I was, experiencing what it would be like to be a teacher with no one to teach, and of course the negative core beliefs of self-doubt predictably arose. But I knew I simply needed to stay with the anxious quiver in the body, say yes to it, and truly feel it.

Once I stayed with the experience for just a minute or two, I felt totally fine about talking to just the one student who had showed up. Interestingly, right at that point, I realized I had the time wrong, and that the meditation session wasn't due to start for another half an hour. But even though many more students (as well as the timekeeper and the attendant) showed up at the right time, it was a very good experience for me to go through. This situation was an opportunity to tap into what is really important to me: to remember that my aspiration is to learn to live from Being Kindness. Once I remembered this, it was no longer an issue whether or not anybody came to see me for a consultation. When we connect with a larger sense of what our life is, negative core-belief thoughts such as "I'll never be appreciated" no longer dictate how we feel and live.

At some point, when that deepest, darkest negative truth about ourselves comes to mind, we have the opportunity to really know that this so-called "truth" is a lie. Only by consciously entering this deep hole inside can we see through these unreal perceptions of who we judge ourselves to be. By breathing the physical feelings right into the center of the chest on the in-breath, we can ultimately connect with awareness of our basic or true nature. This nonconceptual process is how I-as-a-me is transformed into I-as-Awareness. When we truly experience that we are connected with a larger reality, our self-centered reactivity can be included and transformed within the spaciousness of Being Awareness.

As we become more and more familiar with our merciless self-judgments, we can begin to develop a benign tolerance for all of it, even the shame. In looking deeply into ourselves, the qualities of warmth, friendship, and appreciation for ourselves in all of our human foibles begin to come forth naturally. Our self-judgments may still come up, but we will be able to see them through merciful and compassionate eyes.

When we recently boarded a night train between Prague and Kraków, Elizabeth and I were surrounded by a group of pickpockets who pretended to help us with our luggage. At first we didn't know what was happening and we could have easily been robbed. Fortunately, when we realized what was going on, we were able to extricate ourselves from danger. In my earlier years of practice I would have berated myself mercilessly for getting foolishly caught off guard and unaware. This time, instead of slipping into the old pattern of self-judgment, I experienced the entire situation, including my all-too-human "foolishness," with the lightness of Being Kindness.

It's awareness that heals. This is the most fundamental tenet of practice. But for this healing to take place, the depth of our mercilessness must be seen clearly for what it is. Thus, looking deeply is one way of countering our mercilessness of mind.

In addition to basic awareness and knowing our ego's script, there are also specific practices, such as the Being Kindness practices, that can accelerate the process. It takes a certain kind of courage to do this, because the practice of Being Kindness requires that we do something radically different with our core pain of unworthiness, which is to let it in and bring to it the quality of mercy.

Although it's a given that we don't want to feel the pain of unworthiness, at some point we have to understand that it's more painful to hold on to these self-judgments than it is to actually feel them. Mercy is the quality of opening, of allowing the pain to be experienced within the spaciousness of the heart. Mercy is the ultimate yes.

When I first became seriously ill when I was in my late forties, it wasn't yet apparent whether I'd ever get better, and a lot of self-judgment arose around being sick. I believed that if my practice had been deeper, I wouldn't have gotten sick. Moreover, I believed that because I had so much fear around what might happen to me in the future, it proved that I was weak. In fact, there was so much shame, fear, and self-judgment that experiencing these emotions was actually almost as painful as the physical symptoms of my illness.

It wasn't until I started a Being Kindness practice that this mercilessness of mind began to dissolve. The Being Kindness meditation in particular was like an accelerated path, apparently undercutting the solidity of my negative core-belief judgments, including the universal self-judgment of unworthiness. What I learned through the practice of Being Kindness was the real healing, regardless of whether or not my body got better.

We can also learn to bring the quality of mercy to everyday living. We may begin with doing small intentional acts of kindness. But we have to be careful not to get caught in a self-improvement project, trying to make ourselves more kind; even the most virtuous practice can be turned into food for ego aggrandizement. The result is that our efforts will often backfire, and we may end up bitter.

Instead, if we make the efforts with awareness and a little more lightness of heart, often these small acts will bring us face-to-face with our closed-heartedness, which needs to be acknowledged and felt. Yet, regardless of our resistance, we can still make the effort to tap into our innate generosity of heart. Kindness, or generosity, does not have to be obvious, or even overt; sometimes it can just relate to our internal disposition. For example, I fly fairly frequently, and whenever the plane takes off and lands—the times I am told a plane is most likely to crash—I breathe into the center of the chest and bring to mind the people I love the most. The point is to be in conscious connection with my loved ones at the moment of death. But lately I have been making the effort to include whoever I'm sitting next to as well. Sometimes I can even include everyone on the plane. The point is, it's possible for a sense of genuine friendliness to replace the hardness of our normal protective strategies. It's also possible for a real warmth—the warmth of Being-Kindness—to replace our habitual modes of being numb or judgmental.

As we begin to experience a sense of spaciousness around our dark and claustrophobic beliefs of unworthiness, we can discover that there is nothing more satisfying than living from the awakened heart. When we are connected with the Zen Heart, with our true nature, the senses of who we really are and what our life really is are no longer just vague intimations; there is a clarity about what we are doing on this earth, and it is a clarity that brings with it both joy and appreciation.

Perseverence, curiosity, and mercy are three of the most essential qualities in practice. Is one more important than the others? I don't know. Perhaps that depends on where we are in practice. But what is clear is that all three qualities eventually need to be cultivated. In the absence of any one of them, our practice will always be limited.

7

The Three Most Essential Questions

IN THE ME PHASE OF PRACTICE, sometimes it's very difficult to
have clarity when we're caught in the middle of an emotional
upset. This is true even for students who have been practicing
for quite a while. Sometimes, when our emotional drama takes
over, even the most basic practice ideas and techniques go right
out the window.

There's a very common phenomenon—called *cognitive shock*—
that explains why it is so difficult to practice when we're upset.
When we experience distress, the "new" or conceptual brain
tends to stop working. It's as if the shock of distress and the sense
of danger turn off the cognitive mind's basic ability to function. And when the thinking brain is on temporary sabbatical,
we simply can't think clearly. During cognitive shock, the "old"
brain, which is based on survival and defense, takes over. Here,
the primary modes are to attack, withdraw, or go numb, none of
which are conducive to awareness. To be honest, when caught in
cognitive shock, we're fortunate if we can remember to practice
at all!

Even when our brain starts functioning again, we will most
likely take one of the three classic Me Phase detours from reality:
analyzing the situation, thereby taking false comfort in figuring
things out; *blaming* someone or something for our distress, so
that we can avoid feeling it; or *trying to fix* the situation, in order to
take away our discomfort.

We might also get caught in at least one of the three classic inner hindrances: *laziness of mind*, where we don't want to make the effort to look at what's really going on; *self-deception*, where we will maintain the illusions that give us the most comfort; or *self-judgment*, where we are determined to find a flaw in ourselves in relation to what's happening.

And as conditioned beings, we inevitably follow one or more of our characteristic strategies of control when distress hits: *trying harder*, to cover our underlying fears; *seeking approval*, to avoid feeling unworthy; or *escaping or going numb*, to take us away or divert us from the distress we don't want to feel.

When our many detours and strategies obscure the clarity of practice, it is useful to have some concise reminders to bring us back to reality. This is particularly important in the Me Phase of practice, where it is so easy to lose sight of what is most essential. The real question is, what helps us awaken? The answer to this overarching question can be broken down into three very straightforward and specific smaller questions, each of which points us in the direction of clarity.

"Can I Welcome This as My Path?"

This first question—"Can I welcome this as my path?"—is crucial, because if we don't ask it, we're unlikely to remember what practice is. Understanding that our distressful situation is exactly what we need to work with in order to be free is essential. For example, the person we find most irritating may become a mirror—you could call this person "irritating Buddha"—reflecting back to us exactly where we're stuck.

Here's another example: if we're driving behind someone we think is driving too slowly, the practice is to ask, "Can I welcome this as my path?" In other words, can we see this person as our teacher, showing us where we're stuck? In this case, we would be stuck in impatience, in needing life to be different. The same practice applies when someone criticizes us, or crosses us, or when we find ourselves caught in any other emotional reaction or judgment. How quickly do we remember to ask ourselves, "Can I welcome this as my path?"

However, in order to answer this question, we may first need to honestly acknowledge what is happening objectively. We won't be able to use the situation as an opportunity to learn unless we can clearly and objectively see what is actually going on. After all, how can we specifically practice with something if there is a gap between our view of what is happening and the actual fact of the situation?

For example, there's a big difference between thinking (and believing) the thought "She's not very sensitive" and realizing that what is actually happening is that there is a verbal disagreement. Knowing our thoughts helps us see all the judgments we add to the objective data of what is actually going on.

Another example: when we're caught in the swirl of emotional distress, we almost always add the thought that something is wrong. We may think something is wrong in general or, more likely, that something is wrong with another person or with ourselves. In addition, we will almost always add thoughts about how to escape from the distress—through blaming, analyzing, or trying to fix the situation. In short, to effectively work with our emotional difficulties, we first have to clearly see not only what is actually happening, but also what we're adding to the situation, including the detours, escapes, and judgments.

Once, when I was publicly criticized, I felt as if I had been punched in the stomach. My mind almost immediately went into overdrive, justifying myself and blaming the other person. But as soon as I remembered the idea of welcoming the situation as my path, and looked to see what was actually happening (that words had been spoken about me in a public place), nothing of substance remained. The only thing happening in the moment was what I was adding—my reaction of hurt, and the consequent defensive strategy of blaming. There was no objective problem to deal with, in that there was no need to address the critical comments; the only thing I needed to attend to was my subjective emotional reaction. Seeing this allowed me to welcome the experience of hurt and defense as a perfect opportunity to break through the shell of protection—a major step in the Me Phase of practice.

Only when we understand what is actually going on can we make this critical practice step of welcoming our distress. This is where we can literally say yes to it, because we comprehend that as long as we continue to resist our experience, we will remain stuck. So this first question, "Can I welcome this as my path?" reminds us that our difficulties are not an obstacle on the path, but the path itself.

This reminder can't be overemphasized; when we don't remember it, we're likely to fall into hopelessness about practice. We often feel helpless when our usual props break down. This can easily turn into hopelessness and negativity—but this barrier of suffering is only a barrier until we see through it. Seeing through it can lead us to an amazing discovery: that our distress turns into hopelessness only when we forget that it's our teacher. As long as we understand that our situation is an opportunity to learn and grow, hopelessness has a hard time taking root. At this point we may see how our suffering itself can be just another prop, holding together the story of "me."

"What Is My Most Believed Thought?"

The second key question—"What is my most believed thought?"—is one that many skip over, especially since it can be difficult to see what we're really believing. Even though observation of the mind allows us to see our superficial or surface thoughts with clarity, which helps to clear away a lot of the mental story, the most deeply held beliefs often stay below the surface. Thus, the very thoughts that dictate how we feel and act continue to run unnoticed.

For example, our deeply believed thoughts of unworthiness may not be at all on the surface in a given situation; truthfully, in most cases, we may not even be aware of their presence. But their poisonous footprint often manifests itself in our anger, blame, depression, and shame. In fact, such deeply believed and well-hidden thoughts act like radar, seeking out experiences to prove that our beliefs are true. For example, if you believe that you're inadequate, all someone has to do is raise an eyebrow at you, and your radar will tell you you've been exposed for the hopeless mess you believe yourself to be.

Do you know where you get stuck in your own radarlike beliefs? Do you know how to work with them? The practice here begins with asking yourself the question, "What is my most believed thought?"—which is like taking a snapshot of the mind. However, if the answer doesn't come, you drop it, and return to your physical experience rather than trying to figure it out through thinking or analyzing. Then, a little while later, you ask the question again. Sooner or later, with perseverance, the answer will present itself, sometimes with an "aha!"-type quality.

For instance, your surface thought may be, "No one should have to put up with this." This thought expresses the voice of anger and frustration, which we use as a protection. But when we go deeper, a more strongly held thought, such as "I'm nothing," may be revealed with the "aha!" of discovery. Then, as we get to know ourselves, there may also begin to be an "of course" quality. Haven't we seen this belief many times before? It's at this point that we begin to remove some of our investment in our deep-seated core beliefs. But to get to this place, we must first start inquiring into what our most believed thoughts are.

In anticipation of a three-day annual meeting with my peers, I remember being agitated off and on for several days. The surface thoughts kept replaying themselves: "This will be a waste of time," "Nothing ever gets accomplished," and "Why do I want to put myself through this again?" Knowing these thoughts were superficial, I began asking the question, "What is my most believed thought?" At first there was no clear answer, so I returned to the physical experience of mild agitation in the body, specifically the tight chest and the knot in the stomach.

In persevering with the question, the most believed thought eventually presented itself with a crystal-clear quality: "I'm still just passing through." My agitation was the result of my deep-seated pattern of holding myself back, and the subsequent, predictable experience of feeling separate and alone. When I saw what my little mind was believing, it was easier to see that my emotional reaction was founded entirely on what I was adding to the situation rather than on the situation itself; namely, I added judgments about what might happen, judgments based solely on my past conditioning.

The resulting clarity allowed me to reassess my views. This was obviously a perfect situation in which to work with my own Me-stuff, particularly with the feelings of being separate and alone. I then began to welcome the meeting as an opportunity to practice; I even volunteered to host the meeting, so that I could really put myself to the test. It is important to remember that the clarity and subsequent ability to work with this situation were the direct result of asking the question, "What is my most believed thought?" The surprising conclusion was that I even enjoyed the meeting.

"What Is This?"

The third question, which is perhaps the most important, is, "What is this?" As mentioned earlier, this question is the ultimate Zen koan, in that it can't be answered by thinking. The only answer comes from entering directly into the immediate, physical experience of the present moment. Right now, ask yourself, "What is this?" Even if you don't feel any distress, this question can apply to whatever the present moment holds. Become aware of your physical posture. Feel the overall quality of sensations in the body. Feel the tension in the face, particularly around the mouth. Include awareness of the environment—the temperature, the quality of light, the surrounding sounds. Feel the body breathing in and out as you take in this felt sense of the moment. Feel the energy in the body as you focus on the "whatness" of your experience. Only by doing this will you answer the question, what is this?

Admittedly, it is difficult to maintain awareness as we experience the present moment. But it's even more difficult when we're hit with distress, because to truly experience the present as it is means we have to refrain from our most habitual defenses, such as justifying, trying to get control, going numb, seeking diversions, and so on. The sole purpose of these strategies is to protect us from feeling the pain that we don't want to feel; but until we can refrain from these defenses, in both less difficult and more difficult times, we will stay stuck in the story line of "me," unaware of the physical reality of the moment. It's important to understand that being able to ask, "What is this?"—and truly reside with what we find there—takes a great deal of practice and patience.

For example, if we feel anxiety, it's natural to want to avoid feeling it. Maybe we get busy to occupy ourselves, or try harder, or try to figure it out. But if we can ask ourselves the question, "What is this?" the only real answer comes from the actual physical experience of anxiety in the present moment. Remember, we're not asking what it's *about*, which is analyzing—the opposite of being physically present. We're simply asking what it actually is.

When we can truly answer the question, what is this? we will see that our experience, however unpleasant, is constantly changing, and that at bottom, it is a combination of believed thoughts, physical sensations, and old memories. Once we see this, the experience of distress unravels into its individual aggregates, rather than seeming so solid.

As we stay with the question, what is this? we can gradually allow what seems so unpleasant to just be—and reside in the physical experience without attaching all of our emotions, thoughts, and judgments. This is not so easy to do, because our compulsion toward comfort drives us to want to fix or get rid of our unpleasant experiences. To allow our experience to just be often requires that we first become disappointed by the futility of trying to fix ourselves (and others). We have to realize that trying to change or let go of the feelings we don't want to feel simply doesn't work. Staying with the "what is this?" quality of our experience, and allowing it to just be, basically requires a critical practice understanding: that it's more painful to try to push away our own pain than it is to feel it. This understanding is not intellectual but something that eventually takes root in the core of our being.

Once we can really say yes to letting our experience be as it is, awareness becomes a wider and more spacious container, within which distress begins to unravel on its own. The distress may even transform from something heavy and somber into pure, nondescript energy, which is more porous and light. The energy then relaxes on its own, without any need to get rid of it.

The question, what is this? also allows us to bring the quality of mercy or Being Kindness to our practice, because we're no longer judging ourselves, our experience, or others as defective. Instead, we're allowing ourselves to follow an innate curiosity, where we simply want to know the truth of our experience. When we can cease judging, we can begin to experience our life within the spaciousness of the heart rather than through the self-limiting judgments of the mind.

To sum up, these three questions—can I welcome this as my path? what is my most believed thought? and what is this?—remind us of the key steps needed to work with our emotional distress. Some students carry little laminated cards with the three questions in their pockets for times when "cognitive shock" takes hold, when everything we knew about practice is forgotten.

Remember though, these questions are just pointers; take care not to get lost in the technique. The bigger picture of why we ask these questions is that when we have emotional distress, we are usually caught in our own self-imposed prison walls—of anger, fear, and confusion; but when our self-imposed prison walls come down, all that remains is the connectedness that we are. It's important not to lose sight of this bigger context.

Of course, asking these questions, or even remembering them, is based on the most basic question of all: do we want to stay stuck in our emotional distress, or do we want to wake up and be free? The answer to this question is not as obvious as it may seem.

8

The Art of Awareness

I N MY EARLY DAYS as a Zen student, I really wanted to know what it meant to live an awake life. I would often read or hear that "living awake" meant being "one with our experience," so whenever I would meet someone who I thought knew something, I would ask, "What does it really mean to be one with our experience?" I never got an answer that made sense to me, so I began to follow up with the question, "When you're watching a movie, and you're totally absorbed in it, is that the same thing as being one with your experience?" The answer was almost always yes. The absorption experience would usually be equated with being totally in the moment, or awake. Sometimes it was described as analogous to "just chopping carrots," where there is no separation between you and the carrots. Another example was of athletes, who become so absorbed in their activities that they enter "the zone," equating this state of flow with the experience of "no self."

These answers posed a dilemma, since I knew firsthand the experience of being totally absorbed in a movie, which for me was not an experience of being awake. I had also practiced Zen carrot chopping, and had been an athlete who had experienced "the zone" on quite a few occasions—and in none of these instances was I really "awake." Even though there was no sense of self, this no-self experience of being absorbed in activity is often a form of "waking sleep." At best, it's an experience of absorption or concentration. There's nothing wrong with absorption or concentration; in fact, they can foster the enjoyment of artistic creation or athletic performance. However, we can experience these states and still not be truly awake. So to romanticize them with phrases like "being one with activity" is not something that is particularly helpful.

So what *does* it mean to be awake? Along with seeing through the misconception that to be "one with activity" means that we're awake, we also have to abandon the misconception that when we awaken, the experience becomes permanent. Simple observation of ourselves and others would clearly demonstrate that this is untrue. But hope still persists that there is one magical experience that somehow changes us forever. Those who have had powerful "enlightenment" experiences, if they're honest, will admit that even though these experiences may have dramatically affected them, they certainly haven't wiped out their conditioned patterns forever. Quite the contrary, the most pernicious form of waking sleep is believing that we've become an awake *person* just because we were awake for a few moments or hours or even weeks. The diminution of these patterns requires many years of practice in the Me Phase.

Awareness as a Continuum

In actual fact, "awakeness" is a continuum. This continuum does not correspond exactly to the three stages of practice described in this book; rather, the aspects on this continuum interweave throughout each of the different stages of practice. For example, the concentration aspect on the awareness continuum is required in the Me Phase, as well as in the phases of Being Awareness and Being Kindness. Likewise, the wide-open awareness aspect is particularly important in the later phases, but is also relevant even in the Me Phase. The point is, the different modes that are about to be described can be experienced at any time, and are a useful way of gauging to what degree we're awake in any given moment.

On the far end of the continuum, almost as a "pre-stage" to awareness, is the aspect often described as *waking sleep*. This is the state out of which we live most of our lives, although we're often unaware of how asleep we actually are. The single strongest element of this state of waking sleep is that we are *identified*, or lost, in virtually everything—our thoughts, desires, emotions, activities, and so on. More specifically, we're almost always addicted to our thoughts, in that we believe our thoughts and opinions are The Truth. In addition, we can rarely control our emotions; in fact, we often love to indulge them. And perhaps most importantly, we can't stay in the present moment for more than a few seconds at a time. In truth, it's the last place we want to be. Thus, we rarely know who we are or what we're doing, except in a very narrow or self-conscious way. There is no sense of presence or clarity; in a way, we exist primarily as sleepwalkers.

The realization that we're living in this state of waking sleep is often what motivates us to begin practice. Usually, we begin by moving to the *concentration aspect* on the awareness continuum. For example, we may learn to focus intensely on the breath or on sounds. Here we may begin to be "awake," but often only to a very narrow segment of reality. Concentration is not a bad thing—it's just limited, in that it shuts most of life out. However, it's certainly useful in helping the mind and body settle down. If it's done intensely and for a long period of time, it can even set the stage for brief breakthroughs from our normal mode of perceiving reality. For example, in the Zen practice of koan study, our normal bubble of perception may be temporarily broken when the koan is resolved. But the bubble usually closes again quite quickly, and then we're on to the next koan, and the next, possibly ignoring the rest of our life. There may be moments of great insight, but as soon as these moments end, we are likely to become just as angry or fearful as ever.

When practice doesn't bring more awareness and clarity into our everyday life, we may begin to realize that something is lacking. At this point we may become motivated to explore the next aspect on the awareness continuum, which is often called mindfulness. This aspect is particularly relevant in the Me Phase of practice, where we begin to pay more precise attention to our thoughts, emotions, activities, and strategies of behavior. We begin to see clearly the beliefs that run our lives, and the repeating patterns that keep us stuck in our own particular modes of suffering. We also come to know the basic fears out of which all of our beliefs and behaviors arise, and we learn what it means to observe and fully experience our fears without getting consumed by them.

If we persevere with the mindfulness aspect of the awareness continuum, our solid patterns gradually become more and more porous, and our emotional reactions no longer dictate how we live. In this sense, we are, in fact, living more awake. Yet, this is still only one aspect of awareness. We can become very aware of our personal tendencies, and begin to live a more open and genuine life, but still have a very limited awareness of reality.

This is the point where we may realize the need to expand our view of practice even further. As we increasingly understand that practice is not just about nice states of mind induced by concentration or absorption, nor just about freeing ourselves from our personal psychological conditioning, we may move along the continuum of awareness to what is often referred to as *wide-open awareness*. This is the most important aspect in the phase of Being Awareness. In wide-open awareness, unlike the concentration aspect, we are not focused on one particular thing, such as the breath. And unlike the mindfulness aspect, we are not paying as much directed attention to the observation of personal thoughts and feelings. Instead, they may appear and pass like clouds across the sky, and as we become increasingly alert to whatever arises, awareness begins to expand beyond our normal boundaries or limits of perception. This is a very difficult state to describe, but a particular meditation practice, the Three Point Awareness Meditation, opens the door to this expanded awareness state. The instructions for this meditation will be given in the next chapter.

Living Awake

There is a very particular sense—a visceral experience of pres-ence—that can be activated by wide-open awareness. There is a vividness, as if you were "here" for the first time. Sometimes the feeling is almost electric. On occasion, our normal sense of who we are begins to desolidify; and as our fixed boundaries begin to disappear, we feel more connected. We may have the momentary understanding that "all is One" or the equally powerful under-standing that "all is Love"—but those are still only moments. In the actual living of our lives, all of the messy stuff remains. Prob-lems still arise; fear still arises; thoughts still cascade through the mind. The sense of self does not fully disappear, nor does it have to. Yet, something changes. The sense of who we are, the sense of "me," of all my stories, loses its substantiality, its heaviness.

As we begin to relate to the clouds of thought and emotion as just clouds, we no longer feel the need to stop them. They don't go away, but there's a vast difference between identifying with the clouds and identifying with the vast sky within which the clouds appear. Identifying with I-as-Awareness, rather than I-as-a-me, is like identifying with the sky, and from that awareness the clouds are never as substantial as they appear when we're lost inside them. For example, anxiety may arise, but within the wider container of open awareness we can experience the anxiety but not *be* anxious. The narrow sense of I-as-anxious, which normally predominates, gives way to the wider sense of I-as-Awareness.

To live increasingly from the sense of I-as-Awareness, or Being Awareness, is an essential aspect of living an awake life; it is also the direction toward which wide-open awareness practice leads. This is not the narrow experience of absorption, nor of losing our sense of self; rather, there is an experience of awake presence. As awareness expands, as the clouds of attachment and self-centered drama diminish, the experience of living—including the most mundane activities—takes on clarity and freshness. Immersed in activities, there is a *knowing* of who we are—that we are more than just this body, just this personal drama—and the clarity and wonder of our basic connectedness increasingly become a lived reality.

Perhaps the one thing that most prevents us from this awareness is our judgmental mind. It is a readily observable fact that we constantly judge events, ourselves, and others as good or bad. Often, when we have difficult experiences, we automatically make the judgment that something is wrong. And we may then jump to the conclusion that something is therefore wrong with us. This pernicious sense of unkindness often permeates our lives, and consequently prevents us from living in an openhearted and genuine way. Even when we have enjoyable experiences, we often judge them as right and good. Such so-called "positive" judgments do not cause the same suffering as more negative judgments, but they are judgments just the same, and they perpetuate the cycle of waking sleep.

The mindfulness aspect of practice will help us see through our judgmental thoughts to some extent; and the willingness to look with honesty at our unkindness toward ourselves will gradually diminish our self-judgment. Yet, one other aspect of the awareness continuum is essential here: living from the heart of Being Kindness. This is the reason so much emphasis is placed on awareness of the breath into the center of the chest, a practice that has the unique ability to directly undercut the solidity of the judgmental mind. In fact, when awareness is focused in the chest center, it's very difficult to sustain thinking—particularly unkind thoughts. As we direct awareness to this area, the sense of Being Kindness, which is the antidote to self-judgment, begins to come forth naturally. Regardless of how clear we are, or how spacious, without Being Kindness, without a sense of heart, we will surely fall short of living in the way that is most genuine and true to who we really are.

An Analogy

There is a good analogy that describes the kind of awareness required to live more awake. The analogy is to compare the continuum of awareness to a camera. The pre-stage of the awareness continuum, described before as the state of *waking sleep*, where we're basically not aware, not present, is analogous to a camera that still has a dark filter covering the lens. When we begin awareness practice, we are basically learning to take the filter off the lens—we're learning to see and experience in a new way.

The *concentration* aspect on the awareness continuum is analogous to the telephoto lens, where we focus in on one aspect of our experience, such as the breath or a koan, and stay with it very intensely. We also use this lens when we're off the meditation cushion, such as when we need to focus on certain kinds of work, or on creative or athletic endeavors. Here, the concentration aspect may be the most appropriate form of awareness. But when a focused concentration is not required, we change the camera lens to the mindfulness aspect.

The *mindfulness* aspect on the continuum of awareness is analogous to taking a snapshot. With the clarity of a photograph, we examine the present-moment experience of mind and body. We look with precision at the photo, often seeing what we normally might not see, or looking at the same details in a very different way. If there is a strong emotion, we learn how to stay present with the visceral experience of the emotion without getting hooked into the thought-based story—with all of the drama and blame. In *seeing* the thoughts objectively, as we would when looking at a photograph, the thoughts don't fuel the fire of emotion; instead, we can feel the emotion as sheer energy.

When we're using neither the telephoto lens of concentration nor the precise snapshots of mindfulness, we use the wide-angle lens of *open awareness*. The wide-angle lens takes in everything, from the mundane to the shimmering. The experience of wide-open awareness, when the lens is fully open, is like having a 360-degree view while listening to surround sound. There is a *knowing*, a realization, that we *are* the vastness of the surround, as well as a unique manifestation of it. This is the experience of Being Awareness.

What's important to remember is that living awake is not limited to just one point on the awareness continuum. There are times when the telephoto lens of concentration is needed in order to shut out the incessant noise of the mind and to allow the body and mind to settle. There are even more times when the precise snapshots of mindfulness are needed, especially in dealing with our deep-seated conditioning, including all of our emotional reactivity. But as our photo album becomes more and more extensive, as we know ourselves with more and more clarity, we become increasingly capable of including our emotional reactions within the wide-angle lens of open awareness. We learn to experience the clouds while staying with the wide-angle view of the sky. We learn to live increasingly from Being Awareness, able to maintain a larger sense of what life is. And within the spaciousness of wide-open awareness, with the breath centered in the heart, we learn to live each day with Being Kindness as our natural response to life.

Of course, this analogy of the camera lens of awareness is not a scientific formula. But neither is practice. In fact, the attempt to define and confine practice to one thing, or to reduce it to a scientific formulation, is much too limiting. Practice is not science; it is much more of an art form, where we have to deal with the worlds of subtlety, relativity, and paradox. We don't approach all of our experiences with one fixed formula, just as we don't use a camera only one way. Depending on what life is presenting, we learn which lens is needed. In the art of practice, we may flicker between the telephoto lens of concentration, the clear snapshots of mindfulness, and the wide-angle lens of open awareness in a very short span of time.

Truly living awake is even more than an art form; it is ultimately a mystery. But it doesn't have to be mysterious in a confused sense. The more we understand the subtleties of the continuum of awareness, the less we'll be seduced into a single limited view of what living awake means. Rather than seeing it merely as "being one with our experience" or being "mindful" or "spacious," living awake is a fluid interplay of three essential components: a diminution of the self-centered story of "me"; a sense of presence, of Being Awareness; and perhaps above all, the heartfelt sense of Being Kindness that is the essence of who we are.

9

Three Point Awareness Meditation

THE FOLLOWING MEDITATION is a powerful technique for cultivating the state of wide-open awareness described in the previous chapter. As with many meditations it may take some time to become comfortable with the instructions. However, with repeated practice you will find that what at first seemed complicated is actually quite straightforward, and the disciplined effort that's required when learning this meditation later becomes much more natural and fluid.

First Point: Breath into Chest

First take a couple of deep breaths to bring awareness into the body. For this meditation it is best to keep the eyes open and the body still. Bring awareness to the sensations of the breath, particularly the sensations of coolness as the breath enters the nostrils on the in-breath, as well as the subtle texture on the out-breath. Stay with the sensations of the breath in and out of the nose for three full breaths.

Now direct awareness to the feeling of the breath in the center of the chest, feeling the sensations in the area of the heart. On an inhale, breathe *as* if you were breathing directly into the center of the chest, feeling the quality there. Then simply breathe out. Stay with the sensations of the breath in and out of the chest for three full breaths.

Next, direct awareness to the sensations of the belly, feeling the sensations of expansion on the in-breath, and the sensations of contraction on the out-breath. Stay with the experience of the breath in and out of the belly for three full breaths.

Finally, see if it is possible to experience the breath in all three areas simultaneously—the breath in and out of the nostrils, in the center of the chest, and in the belly. You may have to flicker quickly between the three, but place most of the attention on the area in the center of the chest, and stay with this more complete experience of breathing for three full breaths.

When thoughts arise during this part of the meditation, do your best to not get caught in them, and instead keep the awareness focused on the physical sensations of breathing.

As you continue with this expanded experience of breathing, you can also become aware of the rhythm of the breath. Regardless of whether the breath is fast or slow, deep or shallow, regular or irregular, simply notice the rhythm without trying to alter it. Let the breath breathe itself, at its own pace. You don't need to do anything except be aware of it.

As you become aware of the breath's rhythm, be sure to continue staying with the various sensations of breath throughout the body, especially the sensations in the center of the chest. Stay with this expansive experience of the sensations and rhythm of the breath for at least three full breaths.

Awareness of breath, particularly into the center of the chest, is the first point in the Three Point Awareness practice.

Second Point: *Awareness of Environment*

The second point is the awareness of the environment. While still keeping some attention on the breath, bring awareness to the sense of space in the room. You can be aware of the quality of light and the temperature, as well as sounds, including both near and faraway sounds. Simply be aware and listen. There may also be a subtle sound in the head. There may also be sounds between the sounds—the sounds of silence. The sounds don't have to be beautiful—include the traffic, the hum of the refrigerator, the voices of people talking. Simply listen. Listen with the whole body, not just with the ears. As you listen, feel the breath into the center of the chest, while staying tuned to the space around you. Stay with the dual awareness of breath and environment until you can hold the two without too much difficulty. Naturally, attention will wander off repeatedly. The practice is to first return to the anchor of the breath, then to the anchor of the environment, reestablishing the wider container of dual awareness. If possible, maintain awareness of both simultaneously.

If thoughts arise during this part of the mediation, don't push them away. But don't indulge them either. Just notice them, and if necessary, label them to help dis-identify with them. Then come back to the dual anchors of the breath and the environment.

Third Point: Overall Body—"I Am Here"

Once you can hold these two points, attention is directed to the third point, which may be difficult to locate, but which can best be described as the outline of the body. It's the overall feeling of the body-in-space, rather than the directed attention toward any particular sensations. You may want to focus briefly on the tip of the nose, to help you tap into this particular experience of the body. You may also find it helpful to silently say to yourself the phrase "I am here." The "I" in this phrase is not the little "I" of ego but the bigger sense of I-as-Awareness. As awareness expands into this third point, there is a sense of Being Awareness, which is the unique, experiential sense of presence—including the body, yet not limited to the body.

Stay with these three points for the remainder of the meditation, combining awareness of the breath into the center of the chest, the perception of the environment, and the overall feeling of the body. It's perfectly OK to flicker back and forth between them; with practice you'll gradually be able to hold all three at once.

Whenever you drift off into thoughts, here is a crucial instruction: when you become aware that you are caught in thoughts, make the conscious intention to come back to reality for at least three breaths. With the first breath you reestablish the anchor of the sensations of breathing in the center of the chest. With the second breath you reestablish the anchor of the environmental awareness. And with the third breath you reestablish awareness of the overall sense of the body, including the experience of "being here." This particular combination—breath into the chest, awareness of the environment, and awareness of the outline of the body—seems to accelerate the expansion of awareness into the more awake state of Being Awareness.

If you get caught in an emotional reaction during the meditation, you don't need to push it aside. Rather, you just have to temporarily change gears. If the emotion is light, notice and feel it, then reestablish the Three Point Awareness practice. If the emotion is strong, you may need to really focus on experiencing it with "What is this?" mind—which means staying intently present with the physical experience of the emotion. But as soon as the heaviness or agitation begins to lift, move back into the meditation by reestablishing the three points on three successive breaths. It's possible to even include any residue of the emotional experience within the wider container of the Three Point Awareness.

This Three Point Awareness Meditation is the essence of wide-open awareness, where we allow whatever presents itself—

thoughts, feelings, sensations—to arise within the wider container of the three points. Awareness is not limited to just the three points, nor are we staying with the three points in a focused way; rather, we are holding attention to them lightly, and as best we can, continuously. In this way, awareness excludes nothing. This is similar to the Zen practice of *shikan-taza*, with two very important differences. First, the three points give a context within which to experience whatever arises, including thoughts and emotions; and second, they offer a very specific anchor to return to whenever attention wanders. This context and anchor help prevent the practice from becoming amorphous or spacey, which are the major difficulties people sometimes have with shikan-taza. As you develop the ability to maintain the Three Point Awareness practice, it becomes possible, with intention and effort, to tap into this awareness periodically throughout the day, such as during walking, shopping, or driving.

There's an instant version of this meditation that's ideally suited for those moments when you're waiting in line or sitting in your car at a red light. This version emphasizes the phrase mentioned earlier—"I am here." Breathing in, bring awareness to the center of the chest; and on an extended out-breath silently say, "I." On the second in-breath, while continuing to be aware of the breath into the chest center, bring attention to the environment, and on an extended out-breath say, "Am." And on the third in-breath, while keeping the attention peripherally on the breath and the environment, become aware of the overall sense of the body in space, and on the extended out-breath say, "Here." Each word can take on a rich meaning in this brief but powerful exercise. You can do this exercise anywhere, anytime; and as you repeat the three lines, you may instantly enter into the experience of Being Awareness, of living *aware*. Every such moment spent in Three Point Awareness becomes food for one's being.

10
Helpful Daily Life Practices

THE FOUNDATIONS for developing Being Awareness are initially laid in meditation practice, particularly in the Three Point Awareness Meditation, where we move beyond the narrow mind of Me-stuff and enter into a much larger sense of who we are and what life is. Naturally, we also want to bring this more spacious awareness to everyday living, and there are many different tools that can help us with this. For example, cultivating the qualities of perseverance, curiosity, and mercy fosters the ability to shift from our customary identity of I-as-a-me to the less bounded identity of I-as-Awareness. In addition, there are specific practices that can be done in the midst of daily life to facilitate this crucial shift. Three daily practices that I've worked with for many years, and which I still find very helpful, are mapping the mind, gatha walking, and nightly reflection.

Mapping the Mind

Mapping the mind has been around for a long time, and many different versions of it exist. The version presented here is quite simple, yet extremely effective in allowing us to see, from a broader perspective, what runs us. Here's how it works: If you are stuck in an emotional issue, and unclear about what you're actually thinking or feeling, first think of a short phrase that best describes the issue. Then write that phrase down in the middle of a piece of paper and circle it. For example, it could say, "money issue," "relationship difficulty," "depression," or "anxiety over health." Then, over the next few hours or days, whenever a thought, emotion, or strong bodily sensation arises around the issue, write it down on the paper. The entries don't have to be in any order—you can scatter them all over the page.

Basically, you're creating a map of the mind, letting all of the debris that keeps floating through the mind be objectified on paper. In a way this practice is an extended form of thought labeling; but here, we write the thoughts down rather than silently repeating them, and emotions and sensations, as well as thoughts, are included.

It's very important in this exercise to refrain from analyzing the issue. Instead of trying to figure out what's going on, the practice is to objectively observe the thoughts and feelings, then write them down. Don't think too hard about what to write, just let whatever is there pour, unhindered, onto the page. If you start to analyze, you're likely to get even more caught in the spinning mental world—the familiar world of Me-stuff. The point of simply writing the items down is to be able to eventually see with real clarity what you are believing and feeling on both conscious and subconscious levels.

Once you have written down most of the thoughts and feelings (this may take place over the course of a few hours or even days), look at the whole page as if you were looking at a map of your mind. Notice any repeating patterns of thoughts, and also notice the relationship between the thoughts and the emotional and physical feelings. At this point, ask yourself the pivotal practice question: "What is the most believed thought?" There's a good chance the answer will not be apparent immediately, since often the thoughts we write down are superficial or surface thoughts. Repeat this question again, either right away or some time later; if you are intent on knowing what you're believing, the chances are strong that sooner or later the answer will present itself with clarity.

Once the most believed thought becomes apparent, add it to the map of the mind. At this point, when you look at the overall map, it almost always becomes clear how the surface thoughts and also the emotional feelings rose directly from that initial belief. Deeply held beliefs such as "I'll never be appreciated," "I'll always be alone," or "Nothing will ever work out" may sound trite, but their devastating power becomes apparent the more we get to know ourselves.

The point of practicing mind mapping is to be able to see ourselves within a wider container of awareness. When we can see ourselves and our difficult situation with more awareness, we are no longer so identified with the small mind—the mind of I-as-me. The ability to be less identified with our thoughts and emotions is pivotal in being able to live from the more spacious and present place of Being Awareness.

Gatha Walking

I learned gatha walking, a form of outdoor walking meditation, from the Vietnamese Zen teacher Thich Nhat Hanh in the early 1980s, and I've continued doing it (with some lapses) for over twenty-five years. The term *gatha* means "verse," and in gatha walking we silently repeat the gatha as we walk. Unlike affirmations, the gatha is not meant to change our emotional state; rather it is used to direct our attention in specific ways. Gatha walking was once described as the ambrosia of meditations, in part because it requires much less effort than most sitting meditations, but also because it is almost always delightful to do.

The instructions are fairly simple: In an outdoor space, walk at a very relaxed pace, as if you were walking casually through a park. Unlike sitting meditation, where the focus is inward, gatha walking encourages us to engage the senses—seeing, hearing, smelling, touching. To help avoid getting lost in daydreams, we silently repeat a verse, or gatha, over and over. The gatha is usually very short and simple, but the words are meaningful, and help keep the focus on really being here.

The gatha that I've been using for some time has four lines:

> When I walk, the mind will wander.
> With each sound the mind returns.
> With each breath the heart is open.
> With each step I touch this earth.

It is best to repeat the verse for the duration of the walk, even if you start feeling very open and spacious; otherwise, it's easy to become more spacey than spacious. As we walk, we bring awareness to the environment, using the lines to direct our attention. For example, the first line—"When I walk, the mind will wander"—is a way of simply acknowledging the fact that our mind constantly wanders. There's no judgment that the mind's wandering is bad; it's just an objective acknowledgment.

With the second line—"With each sound the mind returns"—we direct attention to the sounds, to help bring us back to present-moment reality. I live close to the ocean, so I have the good fortune to be able to regularly walk along the beach, where I not only use the sounds of the ocean and the gulls but also the presence of wind, the feeling of the sun on my face, the smell of salt water, and whatever other sensory input arises. Being in a beautiful place such as the beach provides a very rich sensory world to take in and appreciate, but we don't have to be at the ocean or in the woods for gatha walking to be a rich experience; I have also had wonderful experiences gatha walking on the busy streets of New York City.

With the third line—"With each breath the heart is open"—we

are not trying to maintain a disciplined focus on the breath. Rather, the breath is very lightly held as it is felt in the center of the chest. Sometimes, it feels as if the breeze goes right through me, with a felt sense that each breath provides food for Being Awareness. With this line, as with the others, we stay with it for the duration of a few breaths before moving on to the next.

On the last line—"With each step I touch this earth"—we can feel the experience of literally walking on the earth, feeling appreciation for the preciousness of the opportunity to be alive. There is an unmistakable sense of presence, of "hereness," that is the essence of Being Awareness.

While gatha walking can be a delightful experience, the purpose of this practice is not simply to make us feel good. In fact, there is no "purpose" in the ordinary sense. In gatha walking, we are not trying to get something, nor are we walking toward a particular destination; rather, each step is complete in itself. Each step is of ultimate value. At the same time, with each step, we are cultivating a much larger sense of what life is.

In our normal walking, with the mind full of thoughts, we see the world only through the filter of our thoughts. In gatha walking, as the mind awakens, the shimmering pulse of life is revealed.

Nightly Reflection

Nightly reflection is a relaxed meditation that is done right before going to sleep. I do it lying on my back in bed with my hands folded on my stomach (this is called the "corpse" position in yoga). The eyes can be open or closed. It's best to do this at approximately the same time each night, and it's especially important to do before getting too tired.

The intention of nightly reflection is to review the events of the day, starting from the first memory of morning to the moment u began reflecting. Focus on the main events, thoughts, and feelings you've experienced throughout the day, as if you were watching the highlights of a movie. During nightly reflection, it's important not to get pulled into thinking and analyzing, but instead to review what actually transpired as objectively as possible, without getting caught in judgments. The instruction is to try to stay physically grounded by maintaining awareness of the breath passing in and out of the center of the chest. Without this grounding, the exercise can easily become too mental.

Once the review is finished, ask yourself two questions: "What am I most thankful for?" and "What do I feel the most remorse for?"

In doing the nightly reflection regularly, we become not only more appreciative during the meditation, we also become more aware and receptive during the day. For example, we begin to notice that we are often not very appreciative as we go through our daily routine. Little positive moments are often not even acknowledged, and then quickly forgotten. But as we become more attuned to what is actually happening during the day, these moments begin to stand out, and we experience genuine appreciation in the present-moment experience.

Similarly, in asking what we are most remorseful for each evening, our sensitivity also becomes much more finely tuned during the day. Interestingly, when we can simply notice, without judging ourselves, where we feel remorse, it is not at all discouraging. In fact, feeling this awakening of conscience is very positive, helping activate the aspiration to live more from the heart. Note that breathing into the center of the chest is particularly important when we are raising these two questions, since it helps avoid the mental detours of thinking and judging.

In effect, by reviewing our day through a focused nightly reflection practice, we're cultivating a bigger container of awareness. Watching the movie clip of the long body of our day allows us to see what we do more objectively, while at the same time being much less identified with it.

During the phase of Being Awareness, a major shift occurs from a focus on I-as-a-me to the less bounded place of Awareness. In order to facilitate this shift, it is often necessary to make conscious efforts, such as those encompassed by these three daily-life practices, in order to cultivate a larger sense of what life is. Mapping the mind allows us to be less identified with our thoughts and feelings; gatha walking helps foster the very tangible experience of being; and nightly reflection helps develop a more expansive perspective while also awakening the essence qualities of appreciation and conscience. Each of these exercises provide food for Being Awareness; and as we slowly (and, perhaps, begrudgingly) drop the story line of "me," the wonder and delight of our basic connectedness increasingly become a natural part of how we live and who we are.

PART THREE
Cultivating Being Kindness

11

Student-Teacher Relationship

As stated earlier, the three phases of practice—the Me Phase, Being Awareness, and Being Kindness—are constantly interwoven throughout the practice life; they do not begin and end at some fixed point. This is particularly true in the student-teacher relationship; yet, the nature and quality of the student-teacher relationship is one of the most important factors in a student's spiritual journey, and will no doubt greatly impact the student's ability to move through the Me Phase and open into the phases of Being Awareness and Being Kindness.

During the course of our spiritual quest it is very common to come to the realization that we need the help of a teacher. Many people don't have a problem with this, but some people never get beyond this barrier. For example, if you don't know you're asleep, it is unlikely that you will look for a teacher to help you wake up. Or, if you view authority with suspicion, believing that it's unhealthy to passively submit to another person, you may never be open to seeking input or guidance. Most of us underestimate how difficult it is for practice to penetrate into the fiber of our being, the fiber of our lives. Not having a teacher compounds this difficulty tenfold. Acknowledging the need for a teacher does not require that you become a true believer or give up your good sense; it does, however, require being open to the fact that you could use assistance. After all, even many teachers still have teachers.

Unfortunately, there's no clear or simple formula for the student-teacher relationship. Each teacher is unique—in temperament, style, and interests. Some are strict and formal; some casual and relaxed. Also, each student is unique. So there's no one particular way the relationship is supposed to be. Even within Buddhism there are three traditional models of the relationship, each quite different from the others; yet they exemplify the most common paths that the student-teacher relationship can take in other traditions as well. In the Tibetan model, devotion to the teacher, who is seen as a guru, is a very important aspect of the relationship. In the Vipassana tradition the teacher is seen as a guide or spiritual friend, quite different from an elevated guru. In Zen the role of the teacher is less defined, although often the teacher is seen as an enigmatic or romanticized agent of transformation, capable of catapulting students into enlightenment with a pointed question or the whack of a stick. Each of these three models has its own merits and its own limitations, but the point is, there is no one way the relationship has to be.

Regardless of the differences in style, the real function of a teacher is common to all: to clarify the basic human problem—that we are disconnected from awareness of our true nature. Individual teachers will approach this differently. One teacher may emphasize the need to leave the thought-based world and enter into the silence of reality-as-it-is. Another may place more importance on the psychological aspect of practice—particularly focusing on the Me-stuff as a way of clearing up clouded perception. And yet another teacher may focus more on specific techniques and meditations to help develop awareness.

Even the same teacher may be understood in different ways by different people. One of my former teachers told me I'm more a Gurdjieff teacher than a Zen teacher. Students sometimes tell me that I seem to teach more Vipassana practices than Zen practices. All the better! No one path can lay claim to the truth. The truth comes in many forms, through many traditions. But regardless of the emphasis taken by any particular teacher or tradition, the point is universal: the need to awaken to our true identity, our basic connectedness.

There are also common stages that a student-teacher relationship will inevitably go through, and in my years as both student and teacher, I've observed three specific stages, each of which can serve as a step toward freedom.

Finding a Teacher

Once we accept the need for a teacher, we have to find one with whom we feel compatible. This may take a period of trial and error, since not every teacher is suitable for every student. In fact, this is where the student's capacity for discernment is very important. Granted that it's difficult to effectively evaluate a teacher on first impression, there are nonetheless some obvious signs that a teacher may not be the best choice. For example, if the teacher speaks with an air of infallibility, or puts other teachers and practices down, or is defensive in response to honest but probing questions, then it might be best to keep looking.

There's one other quality in a teacher that might give us pause. Some teachers are very ready to describe their enlightenment experiences, or perhaps even declare themselves to be enlightened beings, or claim to have the One Truth. Lao Tzu's famous phrase is pertinent here: "Those who know do not say; those who say do not know." Once someone sees themselves as enlightened, any clarity they may have is likely to become delusion. This particular self-deception has been described as one of the most difficult to see through. No one is a finished product, and when teachers see themselves as enlightened beings, they are much less likely to be open to input, particularly when it might go against their self-image as "masters." We need to remember this when looking for a teacher, because there is a part in all of us that would like to be saved by a self-proclaimed enlightened person.

However, also keep in mind that how you feel about a teacher on first impression is not necessarily an accurate way of judging whether a teacher is a good fit. Sometimes our "deepest" feelings, those we usually trust the most, are in fact quite suspect. When I met my first teacher, a teacher in the Gurdjieff tradition, I didn't like him at all. He seemed to be very authoritarian and gruff, and he pushed all my buttons. But I was very committed to the practice, so I stayed with him. Gradually I saw that my initial perceptions were not exactly accurate; as well, I worked with my own reactivity toward him, and came to value his many good qualities.

When I met my second teacher, a Zen teacher, at first I felt I was mostly just passing through, in that I was not committed to either the teacher or the community. For two years I listened to his dharma talks, but rarely understood them—they were full of Zen enigmas, and were more lyrical than practical. But again, I was very committed to the practice, and after a while the talks started to sink in, and I stayed with him for many years.

In short, the search for a good teacher is not always so simple, and trial and error may be the best guideline. However, while trying different teachers in different traditions may be appropriate for a while, we also need to be aware of the possibility that we are playing out habitual patterns of dissatisfaction and doubt or of shying away from commitment. Sooner or later, in order for practice to go deeper, a commitment must be made to one teaching—if not to one teacher. Without this commitment we can never develop the genuine heart connection that is possible in the student-teacher relationship, a connection that feeds our spiritual aspiration in ways that books or words can never do alone.

Difficulties with the Teacher

The second stage in the student-teacher relationship is to learn how to work with the inevitable difficulties that will arise in the relationship. Most often, these difficulties are the result of the student's filters, including all of the expectations and assumptions about what the relationship is supposed to be like. Dealing with these issues in the Me Phase of practice clears the way for our natural Being Kindness to come forth.

One of the most common filters students have is placing the teacher on the proverbial pedestal. The teacher is seen as saintly and wonderful, or more subtly, as the one who knows, unquestionably, what's best. If we come with a childish mind that wants to be saved, we might readily believe the positive projections we then place on the teacher. Of course, when we believe that our teacher "walks on water," we're usually the one who ends up drowning in our disillusionment. This phase in practice, however, is not necessarily a problem; in fact, it can be very valuable when we are forced to face the inevitable disappointment of seeing through this illusion. This phase is only a problem if the student stays caught in it or doesn't know how to practice with the disillusionment of having one's idealized projections on the teacher fall in a heap.

There are other more subtle ways we can place the teacher on a pedestal. For example, you may begin practice with the assumption that the teacher should be perfect, or at least not have certain flaws. You may not be aware of having this obviously unrealistic expectation, but remember, whenever we have a strong reaction to something a teacher says or does, it's a clear indicator that we have the belief that the teacher *should* be different. Take a moment to ask yourself what "flaws" in a teacher aren't OK with you? What is your reaction when the teacher does something you judge as "off"? (Please note that by using the word flaw I'm not talking about conventionally harmful actions.) It's very likely that sooner or later the teacher will do something that will push the buttons on your own personal conditioning. There is guaranteed to be some "flaw" in the teacher that will not only upset you but that will result in you believing your reaction-based judgments as if they were The Truth.

Further, every student, no matter how mature, will bring his or her own ego strategy to the relationship, whether through trust issues, the need to submit to or rebel against an authority, the need to be liked or understood, or something else. Whatever your ego strategy is, it will undoubtedly play itself out in the relationship with the teacher in the same way that it plays itself out in other relationships. For example, if you have an emotional reaction to a difficult situation with the teacher, do you get righteously angry and think you need to speak your mind? Do you withdraw, or feel like giving up? Or do you go numb? It's important to know your own patterns. And it's imperative that you understand what practice entails when these situations occur. First and foremost, you must clearly and honestly see what you are up to. Where might you be imposing your own subjective values? Where might you be reacting from your own blind spots or unseen demands? Where are you repeating patterns that have manifested in previous relationships—patterns that have not yet been addressed?

For example, if you're needy for approval and the teacher is firm in not catering to your ego strategy, you may react from hurt feelings that have little to do with what the teacher is actually saying to you. Ultimately, practice has to entail facing the fears underlying our protective patterns, whether manifested in daily life or in the practice relationship with our teacher. But in order to face these fears, we must first see them clearly. It might also be useful to talk to the teacher about how to best work with the issues that have been triggered. Hopefully, the teacher will be able to help you see what you're doing, even when the teacher and your relationship become part of the subject matter.

We have so many uninvestigated assumptions about teachers that they are bound to cause us difficulties at some point. Why? Because teachers aren't perfect; and they, like their students, are engaged in an ongoing process. In fact, unless teachers continue to work at their own edge and with their own fears, they will become disconnected from others, and thus lose their effectiveness as teachers.

Teachers, perhaps more than anyone, have to be honest with themselves; they have to be willing to see their own limitations. For example, a naïve student may want to believe that the teacher is a mind reader, but a teacher can never know with certainty how a teaching will be taken by a given student. The Dalai Lama spoke about an elderly monk who came to ask him whether he thought it would be good for him to do hatha yoga. The Dalai Lama told him that maybe he was too old to begin such a physical endeavor. Later the Dalai Lama heard that the monk had committed suicide, in the hope that he could be reborn in a younger body capable of doing yoga! How could the Dalai Lama have known that his straightforward advice would lead to this sad result? In this sense there is no blame, yet a teacher will still feel the weight of events such as these.

Of course, there are certain situations when the teacher may, in fact, act inappropriately. It may not be an obvious problem, such as having sex with students, taking money inappropriately, or abusing alcohol or drugs, but it may still need to be addressed. Apart from these obviously inappropriate situations, the focus here is on the more harmless interactions that cause us to react. And the main point is that it's best to work with and see through our own emotional reactions first, because most of our reactions are based on our own assumptions and conditioned views. For example, there is a common assumption among students that the student-teacher relationship is supposed to be pleasant, or at least not difficult. If this assumption is on board, there will surely be a reaction when the teacher points to something in you that you hadn't noticed and perhaps don't want to see. Likewise, if you expect the relationship to be easy, how will you react when you're asked to practice with something that you're unwilling to practice with? But if you only do what makes you feel comfortable, or what is easy, you become less and less open to learning. This is unfortunate, because even the most skillful teacher can teach only in proportion to the student's willingness to learn.

When you realize what assumptions and agendas you bring to the relationship, it doesn't mean you should beat yourself up for your "faults," or struggle to be a better student. What it does mean is that you can become increasingly aware of your own beliefs and actions, using them and the difficulties they create in the student-teacher relationship to go deeper in your practice. The point of being a student, after all, is to learn. And it is the wish of every teacher to see students learn to stand on their own two feet, and to become free of their conditioned beliefs and behaviors. The less we act out of our agendas, particularly our dependence on an authority, the more we can be who we truly are. From that place, we can live from the Being Kindness that is our natural essence.

Standing on Your Own Two Feet

As stated, one part of the teacher's job is to help students clarify their individual difficulties, including each student's particular conditioning and set of hidden beliefs. On this level the teacher has to work very individually and specifically with each student, since some students, for example, may have a great deal of anger, while others have more fear or confusion.

Sometimes, especially in the early years of practice, the teacher may actively support the student, helping to carry the student in a way, until the student develops the discipline necessary for practice to mature. Later, as the student's practice evolves, the teacher may say very little. At a certain point, by simply being heard, or asked pointed questions, the student will feel encouraged to stay on the path.

Given the teacher's job, it might be easy to mistake the teacher's function. The function of the teacher is certainly not to be the student's substitute parent. Nor is it to be the student's therapist, even though the practice will often include working on the psychological level. This is a tricky point. The fact that we are psychological beings can't be ignored, which means we have to learn to work with our anger, fears, and strategies of protection. But the point of this work is not simply to understand ourselves better, or "improve" ourselves in order to live in a more stable and comfortable way. This may be the point of traditional psychology, but in spiritual practice we are learning to be with ourselves as we are, with life as it is, and to become free from the narrow, constricting, and artificial concepts of "me" as a separate self. It is the function of the teacher to point students in the direction of that freedom. All of the teacher's techniques are ultimately geared to allowing students to see through their illusory constructs, in order to awaken to their true nature.

As students, we have to recognize that there are many things we don't know. Much of the Me Phase of practice is about deepening our knowledge of ourselves, our "me." Even after moving out of the Me Phase, there will still be a great deal to learn. But when we enter the phase of Being Awareness, a different type of learning takes place. We learn to expand beyond our customary perceptual filters—filters that seem to fall away naturally in practices such as the Three Point Awareness Meditation. We can then begin to connect with a larger sense of what life is.

As we move outside the boundaries of the familiar—boundaries that ordinarily help us survive and make sense of things—we will most likely encounter fear, especially fear of the unknown. Here the teacher's role is crucial. At this point the teacher's task is to help the student stay present with his or her experience of seeming groundlessness—an experience that is likely to be difficult and sometimes even terrifying. A teacher who has been through the process can encourage the student to keep going, to not turn away from the spaciousness of Being Awareness even when the experience is frightening. Through this process, students develop a deepened sense of trust in themselves and in the practice.

The teacher's role in the phase of Being Kindness is equally important. Here the teacher may encourage the student directly with words, but also indirectly, by example. For instance, when a teacher doesn't judge a student, regardless of what the student brings up, the student learns that it's possible to live without judging, either others or ourselves.

When the teacher can truly teach from Being Kindness, students will be inspired to go deeper in their own practice. What they originally saw as good qualities in the teacher, such as clarity and kindness, they now see as a reminder of and reflection of what is also present inside themselves. Both from the teacher's words and example, students can gradually develop a basic trust in themselves—in the Being Kindness that is their own true nature.

In a way, everything a teacher does is ultimately directed toward helping students awaken to their true nature. This is what allows students to develop independence, to stand on their own two feet, no longer even needing the regular guidance of their teacher. It is unfortunate that some teachers require their students to remain dependent on them, because truly living from Being Kindness should ultimately never be dependent on another, even one's teacher. Living from Being Kindness is only dependent on awakening to who we really are.

Does this mean that at some point we no longer need a teacher? The answer is a qualified yes. It's qualified because we may make the choice to stand on our own before we are ready. I have even seen excellent teachers with deep clarity fail to recognize, at certain points, the emergence of elements of their own Me-stuff. They could still function as good teachers, but because their learning process, particularly the ability to see their own blind spots, was impeded by being solely on their own, they never learned to truly live from Being Kindness. As a consequence, they remained, at least partially, stuck in their own conditioning.

Suffice it to say that none of us are ever beyond the need for input on occasion, which is why the most effective teachers are those who remain receptive to learning and who exemplify humility in their unknowing. However, it is in fact possible to stand on our own two feet, provided we have become unrelentingly honest with ourselves, combined with the pivotal understanding that when we really pay attention, *everything* is our teacher.

12
Transforming Anger

MANY PRACTITIONERS get discouraged when they realize how difficult it is to maintain an awake state. Quite often, even after a good period of meditation or yoga first thing in the morning, where we feel somewhat aware and awake, we may "come to" later in the day with the realization that we've since spent hours in a state of waking sleep. The question is, why is it so hard to awaken? In part, it's because the life force, or energy, necessary to awaken is constantly leaking away, from morning till night.

Perhaps the most significant leak occurs through the manifestation of negative emotions, where energy is squandered in small and sometimes huge doses throughout the day. The word *negative*, as used here, doesn't necessarily mean "bad," but simply something that negates or denies. It says no to life. Anger, for example, says, "I don't want this!" This does not apply only to loud outbursts of anger. We manifest negative emotions, in smaller doses, all day long: as irritability, judgments of self and others, impatience, passive aggression, and so on.

Working with Anger

One important emphasis in practice is learning what closes these leaks. This is why we must pay attention to how to work with our negative emotions, particularly the many forms of anger. An analogy might be helpful in understanding this process: we all know that food provides energy for the body. But there's another kind of "food" that feeds our being, namely our impressions or experience. Every experience, much like the food we consume, can either nourish or deplete us, depending on how much awareness is present and what our intention is. When we react to an experience negatively, it's like eating bad food. It doesn't digest. In fact, it can even poison us. When that happens, we often spew the poison back out into the world, usually at another person.

The alternative to manifesting negative emotions is to bring physical awareness to the actual energy of the reaction. Normally, we fuel our reactions by believing and justifying the thoughts that accompany them. But when we disengage from this pattern, attention can instead be focused on the visceral experience of the emotion itself. This attention allows a different type of digestion to take place. For example, when we can stop the *expression* of anger and instead *experience* its actual energy, that raw energy may actually transform into nourishment for Being Awareness.

I'm not suggesting that emotions should not arise, nor that we should repress them. The practice instruction is simply to refrain from *expressing* them, either outwardly through words and actions or inwardly through spinning and obsessive thoughts. It is only through the process of not expressing negative emotions and instead actually experiencing their energy that we learn to live in accord with our true nature, our natural Being Kindness.

If we could see our angry emotional reactions clearly, it would become obvious how they deplete our energy and consequently narrow our life. We would also see how, when we're caught in anger, we're cut off from the heart, from a sense of our basic connectedness. For example, when someone swerves in front of us on the freeway, anger arises instantly, and we may get caught in the strong impulse to yell and gesture. We will certainly feel justified in being irate. But what happens if, instead of expressing the anger, we simply stay with the visceral experience?

Practicing in this way over time teaches us to connect more deeply with our experience, and finally we are able to recognize the situation as it is: that another driver simply cut us off, and that is all. Perhaps we can also label the reactions we have as just believed thoughts, such as, "Having a believed thought: 'he's a moron,'" "Having a believed thought: 'she shouldn't be allowed to drive,'" or "Having a believed thought: 'this always happens to me.'"

As we learn to see our reactions more clearly, and to label the thoughts associated with them, we become more and more capable of experiencing our anger as just what is—heat in our face or tension in our muscles and gut. We might even see that what really happened is that we simply got scared. Above all, we no longer hold on to our emotions and thoughts as the objective truth about what actually happened.

At a certain point, in addition to experiencing our emotions and labeling our thoughts, we may even feel compassion—in this example, for the driver who cut us off—or at least we might laugh at ourselves for getting so worked up over an objectively small or insignificant occurrence. The point is, when we don't express anger, not only is the energy leakage closed, but the very energy that would have leaked away also becomes available for nourishing a genuine reconnection with life.

One common point of confusion relating to this process is misunderstanding the difference between nonexpression and suppression. When anger is suppressed, it means that we are not feeling it. This can be particularly problematic for meditators who have been brought up suppressing their anger, because they can easily mistake their suppression for spiritual maturity. But suppressed anger tends to fester; the poisonous energy of anger can even pollute the body, often impacting our physical health. When we instead withhold the expression of anger, it is very different from suppression. Nonexpression actually allows us to feel—to fully feel—the emotion of anger directly, letting it simply be there without needing to do anything about it.

So why is it so difficult to stop the expression of anger? We seem to hold on to this habit with a stubbornness that defies all sense. The simple answer is we *want* to be angry. We want to be right. This may not always be obvious, but the feelings of juiciness and power that can accompany the expression of anger are often intoxicating. This makes sense from an evolutionary point of view, where raw instinctual reactions served a real purpose— they allowed us to ward off physical threats in order to survive. However, even though we no longer face the same kinds of danger, and thus no longer need the same kind of response, our bodies and minds have not yet caught on. So that juicy, "good" feeling of anger remains, though it no longer serves us, particularly if we are on the path of trying to live a more harmonious life.

There is another important reason why we may choose to stay angry. Expressing negative emotions can cover over the fear-based pain that often underlies our anger—the pain that we simply don't want to feel. For example, we will often feel an immediate surge of anger when we are criticized. Most of the time, we will jump directly into blaming and self-justifying, which is our automatic defense mechanism or protective strategy for avoiding feeling the pain of rejection and unworthiness that the criticism triggers.

But if instead we refrain from expressing anger, we can go deeper into our experience and truly feel not only the energy of anger itself but also the core of pain beneath it. This is often a quiet inner process, where we stay intently present with our experience in a way that allows us to break through layers and layers of protective armoring. We thereby enter into the fear-based pain we've never wanted to feel; and while it is certainly not pleasant to be with our most deeply seated pain and fear, it is only by uncovering and residing in this place that true transformation can occur. Only here can we ultimately reconnect with our basic wholeness.

I've been doing a practice for the last fifteen years that has helped me tremendously in working with anger. The practice is called the Nonmanifestation of Negative Emotions. I do this practice one full day a week, starting first thing in the morning and continuing until I go to sleep. The practice involves making a conscious effort not to manifest any negative emotions for the entire day, through either external behavior or internal ruminations. This does not mean, however, that anger and other negative emotions will not arise, because surely they will. What it does mean is that as soon as we become aware of them, we make the conscious effort to refrain from indulging the thoughts that fuel those particular emotions.

Again—and I cannot stress this point enough—this practice is not about emotional suppression, nor about trying to modify our behavior in order to become a better person. This practice is about awareness. Because we are particularly alert on the day we choose to do this practice, we will often catch the emotion at its inception. Furthermore, we will be less likely to be caught off guard by our reactions. And when anger and other negative emotions do arise, it becomes increasingly possible to choose to turn away. We can make this choice because the emotion has not yet solidified, nor has it begun to gather energy fueled by the believed thoughts that usually accompany the emotion.

Essentially, this one-day practice allows the identification with "me" and "my emotions" to fall away. As this happens, we open to the more spacious sense of I-as-Awareness. It's actually quite amazing to see how easy it can be not to indulge our anger; it is equally amazing to truly realize the extent to which we *want* to be angry. There comes a point where we can see that we don't have to indulge that desire, and that our anger is almost always optional. Granted there are times when anger may arise very strongly, and it may not then readily dissolve with our choice not to indulge it. But if we make the effort to not let our thoughts get a toehold, and stay focused on the physical energy of the emotion itself, the anger will often dissipate quickly.

Even if the anger doesn't dissipate, we'll at least have a very good chance of bringing awareness to the root of it. Usually we're so caught in the mushroom-cloud explosion of anger that there is little awareness of the fear out of which the anger arises. In the earlier example of being cut off on the freeway, by declining to express or fuel the angry reaction, we're more likely to see that what the incident first provoked was fear, and how, as a protection, we immediately moved into anger, probably without even being aware of the fear.

It's very important to persevere with the practice of Non-manifestation of Negative Emotions throughout the day, especially after those inevitable moments when anger catches us off guard. Here, instead of judging ourselves as bad practitioners and giving up, the practice is to simply take a breath into the heart and extend Being Kindness to ourselves. The element of lightheartedness is absolutely necessary to keep this one-day practice from becoming just another grim fix-it project.

As long as we keep coming back to the original intention and reminding ourselves that the purpose of this practice is awareness, we may make the wonderful discovery that we don't have to express our anger whenever it arises, nor do we have to justify it by defending our believed thoughts. Instead, we can learn that it's possible to live increasingly from the spaciousness of Being Awareness and the heart of Being Kindness, rather than from the dark and narrow identification with "me"—and an angry me at that.

Until we learn to refrain from expressing anger, and instead experience it, we will keep wondering why the life force that is so necessary to awaken eludes us. Realizing this, however, is not a conceptual process; no amount of thinking will allow us to understand what is at work here. The only way of really verifying the truth of this transformative process is to stop the habitual mode of expressing and justifying anger when it arises. This is crucial if we are to wake up.

Anger as Resolve

Sometimes anger arises so quickly that it takes over before we're even aware of what's happening. As a countermeasure, we can ask the three essential practice questions. First, as soon as we acknowledge that we're angry, we ask, "Can I welcome this as my path?" Next, in order to see all of the expectations and requirements out of which our anger arises, we ask, "What is the most believed thought?" And last, we ask, "What is this?"—truly feeling the energy of the anger and letting it just be.

However, sometimes our anger feels so strong that even asking the practice questions won't help. Sometimes the thoughts are so unrelenting, particularly the blaming thoughts, that we have to take stronger measures. One practice I find useful, when thoughts of blame and self-justification become obsessive, is to say the phrase "Don't go there!" Whenever the predictable thoughts recur, I repeat this phrase until the obsessive cycle loses steam.

Once, when I was struggling with a very powerful bout of anger, Elizabeth walked into the kitchen where I was cooking and asked me who I was talking to. It turns out I was actually saying "Don't go there!" out loud! We both got a laugh out of that, although usually it isn't funny at all when anger takes over. In fact, doing this practice in the midst of feeling angry requires a definite assertion of will, grounded in a strong intention not to indulge the angry thoughts. But over time, as the obsessive cycle weakens, we can return more and more easily to the three essential practice questions.

With meticulous practice, strong anger can even bestow a useful gift. As the energy of anger is worked with, it can transform into resolve, helping us carry through with appropriate action in situations that require a response. Unfortunately, it is much more common to justify our actions through anger well before we have really worked with the situation internally. The danger here is that we act from the negative energy of anger, but from the point of view of spiritual practice, there is *never* a justification for visiting the poisonous negativity of anger on another, no matter how righteous we may feel.

When we act from anger, we make life the enemy, along with everything in it, whether that be a person, a group, or even a country. In this stance, we are deeply caught in the narrow place of I-as-a-me, where we have lost all contact with our basic connectedness. However, when this narrow sense of "me" is included in a wider container of awareness, we can avoid following the painful and seductive path of self-righteousness. With awareness, it is possible to experience the energy of anger without getting hooked into the story line of its thoughts.

As the energy of anger transforms into a sense of purpose and resolve, minus the usual negative overlay of anger itself, we may engage in life with both clarity and an open heart. There is no longer an enemy, just the desire to live from what is most genuine within us. There is the example of Gandhi, who was once about to lead a very large peaceful march to protest the British policy on harvesting salt from the sea. Thousands of his followers were waiting to begin the march, but when Gandhi realized how much anger was still in his heart, he went off to meditate and work with his anger. He was willing to let his followers wait and deal with all the practicalities of waiting rather than act precipitously from anger. Days later, he emerged and was ready to begin the march—no longer focused on the British as the enemy but instead filled with a sense of peace, clarity, and purpose.

I don't mean to make the transformation of anger sound simple or easy. My own experience has taught me how difficult this can be. When I joined my first spiritual group, they used to call me the Prince of Negative Emotions. My own children used to call me the Black Cloud when they were young, in reference to those times that my anger would fill up our entire household. Often I didn't even know how angry I was until someone pointed it out to me. That's why acknowledging anger is always the first step in practicing with it. As I became more and more familiar with the many faces of my anger, it gradually became clear to me how much pain I was causing, both for myself and others. Even knowing that, as I persevered in working with my own anger, I would still sometimes watch myself get totally caught in it in spite of everything I knew. But when discouragement threatened to take over, I slowly learned to bring Being Kindness to my all-too-humanness, and I never gave up.

Now, many years later, anger does not arise very often, and when it does, it rarely sticks. But there are still those times where I can see anger trying to take over, especially when I feel within me the familiar seductive juiciness of wanting to indulge it. What I have found most helpful is to invoke a particular phrase that reminds me of my aspiration to live from the heart. When I catch the anger arising, I ask the question, "What would it mean, in this very moment, to live from Being Kindness?" When I reflect on this question before speaking or taking action, the considered response is almost always to turn away from the painful and separating negativity of anger.

For example, one evening Elizabeth and I had a disagreement right before going to sleep, and as I was lying there on my back, I felt myself caught in wanting to be right, including the small-minded wish to punish her by not turning over and curling up with her, as is our custom. But when I remembered to ask myself, "What would it mean, in this very moment, to live from Being Kindness?" I immediately turned on my side to feel her next to me, and in that instant all the anger dissolved. In this case, just asking the question was all that was required. Our anger may not always dissipate as quickly as it did in this situation, but just asking the question made it clear to me what was most important.

Asking and reflecting on this question is not about trying to live from ideals, but rather a way of invoking the aspiration to live genuinely from the heart; if our words or actions don't come from Being Kindness, why would we want to take them? In the third phase of practice, where we're learning to actually live from Being Kindness, this intention becomes the context that guides us. Then, even our anger can become the path to living from the heart.

Blaming and Forgiveness

When we feel that others have hurt us, our usual tendency is to judge and blame them. We are also rarely aware that our blaming is mainly an attempt to cover our own pain, including the pain of seeing ourselves as diminished, or as not enough in some way. So we get angry or resentful, and then focus on the shortcomings of those who have hurt us.

But in our blaming there is another subtle dynamic going on. When we take offense at others, we think our offense or hurt is the result of what they did or didn't do. We thus use their behavior to justify our anger. In so doing, we're missing a crucial point: when we get caught in blame and justification—in our anger and resentment—we have lost our own way. We have cut ourselves off from the heart, from the love and connection that are our true nature.

While some situations may, in fact, eventually require taking objective steps to remedy potentially harmful outward actions, the real transformative process is an inner one. We have to acknowledge that it is our own darkness that has pulled us off the path, not the darkness of the other. Even though the other may have done something unskillful or unkind, this never justifies our unkindness in return.

Though something in us already knows this, it often takes only a nanosecond to go from this innate understanding to the mental realm of judging and blaming the other. Sadly, it is from our own unkindness toward the other, as manifested in our judging and blaming, that we make the choice to live from a closed heart. And in so doing, we are choosing to live as a victim, insisting on being right and elevating ourselves by putting the other down.

The question remains, why do we do this? In part, it is because we live out of two equally false self-images: One is the negative belief that at our core we are nothing, that we are fundamentally unworthy. The other is the compensatory self-image, such as being kind or worthy, that we develop in order to cover over the negative one. Neither of these images is the truth; they are merely two sides of the same delusion. And as long as we live out of these self-images—rooted in the syndrome of unworthiness—and as long as we continue to blame others out of fear, or the need to elevate ourselves, we solidify the ego identity of I-as-a-me. In so doing, we continue to disconnect from ourselves, from our natural Being Kindness.

Practicing with anger ultimately allows us to see that when people treat us unkindly, it is their action, born of their suffering, and has little to do with us. And while we may still want to use their actions to justify our negative reaction, we should be aware that we have another choice; we can instead choose to turn away from blaming. When we can, in fact, turn away from blaming—which entails a willingness to feel our own anger, hurt, and fear—we open ourselves to relating to the other in a new way. We are now able to see them in their all-too-human garb, as just another human being in pain. Perhaps we may even understand that they were not trying to hurt us, but simply acting out of their own pain-induced closed-heartedness.

For example, suppose we feel hurt by someone's words or actions. The ego will react almost immediately with anger and righteousness. The usual defenses, such as self-justifying and blaming, will arise from the fear of feeling unworthy and from the attempt to posit a strong image. No one wants to feel the hurt or fear, so we use this shield of anger to protect ourselves. We might fall into the righteous mode—making our case, being right. We might elevate ourselves by subtly putting the other down, one of the surest signs that we're acting from the small mind of insecurity. But in so doing we're ignoring whatever our part may have been in triggering the hurtful words or actions. We have to remember that when difficulties such as these arise between adults, no one is totally blameless; at times, we all do things that are potentially harmful. We may know somehow that we are ignoring the unkindness we've perpetrated against the person we perceive as hurtful, but because we do not want to acknowledge our own unkindness, we may try to write it all off as the other person's fault, to justify our anger. Yet, if we look more closely inward, we may realize that our anger is being used, at least in part, to avoid feeling remorse for our own insensitivity to the other.

But even if we didn't mistreat the other, we can still be caught in the stance of righteous blaming. With this mind-set, we're cutting ourselves off from living from our true nature. Yet, when we can stay with our visceral experience, without defending, we may truly see our own unkindness. We may also clearly see the unkindness of the other for what it really is: the unskillful act of someone in pain.

Working with anger and other negative emotions in this way is not easy; we simply do not want to move away from blaming because that exposes us to pain. But when we can honestly experience our own pain without blaming others for it, we can truly begin to see the other's struggle as no different from our own. As we become aware of not only our own pain but also that of another human being, genuine compassion for ourselves and the other can arise naturally. And from this place, there is really no one to forgive, because the sense of separateness, of "I" forgiving "you," is no longer operative. In its place is the heartfelt connection with another that comes when we can see them with real clarity, no longer blinded by our emotional neediness and reactivity.

When we refrain from judging and blaming, we have an opportunity to cease our unkindness toward others (regardless of their unkindness toward us) and to experientially reconnect with the heart. When we truly abandon our blaming and *see* that we have not been hurt by others but by ourselves, and likewise that they are not hurting us but themselves, genuine compassion and forgiveness come forth without effort. And when our equanimity is no longer dependent on how others treat us, we are inwardly free to live from the Being Kindness that is our true nature.

13

The Things We Fear Most

WHEN THINGS UPSET US, we often think that something is wrong. Perhaps the one time this is most true is when we experience fear. In fact, as human beings, a huge portion of our energy is expended in dealing with anxiety and fear. Fear motivates how we act and react, and even how we dress or talk. But fear makes our life narrow and dark. It is at the root of all conflict, underlying much of our sorrow. Fear also blocks intimacy and love, and, more than anything, disconnects us from the Being Kindness that is our true nature.

Even considering how prevalent fear is in our lives, it nonetheless remains one of the murkiest areas to deal with, in daily life as well as in practice. This may sound bleak, but what is really the worst thing about fear? Though it may be hard to admit, especially if we see ourselves as deeply spiritual, the main reason we have an aversion to fear is that it is physically and emotionally uncomfortable. Woody Allen put this quite well when he said, "I don't like to be afraid—it scares me." We simply don't want to feel this discomfort, and will do almost anything to avoid it. But whenever we give in to fear, we make it more solid, and consequently our life becomes smaller, more limited, more contracted. In a way, every time we give in to fear, we cease to truly live.

The question remains, what are we so afraid of? Think for a minute about the two or three things you fear most. Keep your answers in mind as you read the following pages, so that your reading can be more experiential than intellectual.

We're often not aware to what extent fear plays a part in our lives, which means that the first stage of practicing with fear requires acknowledging its presence. This can prove to be difficult, because many fears may not be readily apparent, such as the fear driving our ambition, the fear underlying our depression, or perhaps most of all, the fear beneath our anger. But the fact is, once we look beyond our surface emotional reaction, we will see that almost every negative emotion, every drama, comes down to one or more of the three most basic fears—the fear of losing safety and control, the fear of aloneness and disconnection, and the fear of unworthiness.

Security and the Loss of Control

The first most basic fear is that of losing safety. Because safety is fundamental to our survival, this fear will instinctually be triggered at the first sign of danger or insecurity; the old brain, or limbic system, is inherently wired that way. This particular fear will also be triggered when we experience pain or discomfort. But in most cases, even when this fear is triggered, there is no real danger to us; in fact, our fears are largely imaginary—that the plane will crash, that we will be criticized, that we're doing it wrong. Yet, until we see this dimension of fear with clarity, we will continue to live with a sense of constriction that can seem daunting.

Once we become familiar with our insecurities, a central component of spiritual life is recognizing that practice is not about ensuring that we feel secure or comfortable. It's not that we won't feel these things when we practice; rather, it's that we are also bound to sometimes feel very uncomfortable and insecure, particularly when exploring and working with our darker emotions and unhealed pain. Yet, there is also a deep security developed over the course of a practice life that isn't likely to resemble the immediate comfort we usually crave. This fundamental security develops instead out of the willingness to stay with and truly experience our fears, which means to enter into the *physical* experience of fear itself—the racing heart, the contractions in the chest and belly, the rigid face muscles, the hormones coursing through the body. Isn't it ironic that the path to real security comes from residing in the fear of insecurity itself?

Insecurity can also manifest as the fear of helplessness, often surfacing as the fear of losing control, the fear of being controlled, the fear of chaos, or even the fear of the unfamiliar. For example, nearly all of us have experienced the emotion of rage, which is like being swept into a mushroom-cloud explosion. Think of all those days where nothing seems to go your way, or even just the last time your TV remote stopped working, and no matter what buttons you pushed, you couldn't get it to do what you wanted. The urge to throw the remote against the wall can feel like angry rage, but as we bring awareness to this experience, we can discover that the feeling of rage is often just an explosion covering over the quieter inner implosion of feeling powerless. Rage may give us a feeling of power and control, but how often is it an evasion of the sense of powerlessness that feels so much worse?

We all dread the helplessness of losing control; yet, real freedom lies in recognizing the futility of demanding that life be within our control. Instead, we must learn the willingness to feel—to say yes to—the experience of helplessness itself. This is one of the hidden gifts of serious illness or loss. It pushes us right to our edge, where we may have the good fortune to realize that our only real option is to surrender to our experience and let it just be.

During a three-year period in the early 1990s when I was seriously ill, with no indication that I would ever get better, I watched my life as I had known it begin to fall apart. I not only lost my ability to work and engage in physical activities but also experienced a dismantling of my basic identities. At first, it was disorienting and frightening not to have the props of seeing myself as a Zen practitioner, a carpenter and contractor (my livelihood), a husband and a father. But as I stayed with the fears, and particularly as I was able to bring the quality of Being Kindness to the experience, there came a dramatic shift.

As the illusory self-images were stripped away, I experienced the freedom of not *needing* to be anyone at all. By truly surrendering to the experience of helplessness, by letting everything I clung to just fall apart, I found that what remained was more than enough. Naturally, as I got better, my identities tried to put themselves back in place, but, like Humpty Dumpty, the protective cocoon of a "me" would never be quite the same. As we learn to breathe fear into the center of the chest, the heart feels more and more spacious. I'm not talking about the heart as a muscle in our chest, but rather the heart that is our true nature. This heart is more spacious than the mind can ever imagine.

Aloneness and Disconnection

The second basic fear is that of aloneness and disconnection, which can also manifest as the fear of abandonment, loss, or death. On some very basic, yet very deep level, all of us feel fundamentally alone; and until we face this directly, we will fear it.

It's interesting that one of life's most vital lessons is something we are never taught in school: how to be at home with ourselves. When I first began going to meditation retreats, where there was no talking or social contact for days on end, I would sit facing the wall hour after hour, and invariably an anxious quiver rose up inside me. Sometimes it was so strong that I literally wanted to jump out of my skin. But just sitting there, doing nothing, brought me face-to-face with myself, with my fear of aloneness.

Most people will do almost anything to avoid this fear. Many enter into relationships or engage in affairs. In fact, the extent to which people have affairs is often proportional to the urgency of needing to avoid feeling alone. Ultimately, however, the willingness to let loneliness just be—by truly residing in it—is the only way to transcend it. It's also the only way to develop true intimacy with another, because true intimacy can't be based on neediness or on the fear of being alone. When we need people, we can't truly love them, because we will see them and relate to them through the small mind's filter of neediness.

Still, we want and expect other people to take away these fears; we think that if we're with someone who will pay attention to us, our loneliness will disappear. But if this particular deep-seated fear is part of our makeup, the mere act of our partner being engrossed in a book when we're expecting attention will be enough to make us feel abandoned. We may try to deal with this by demanding or attempting to attract their attention, but even if that demand is met, our fear is unlikely to be assuaged for long.

Furthermore, even getting the attention we desire does not necessarily mean we will experience intimacy. True intimacy comes instead when we're willing to acknowledge the uncomfortable feelings of anxiety and fear that are part of our own conditioning; it comes when we can say yes to them, when we can breathe the aching longing of loneliness into the center of the chest and simply let it be there, no matter how uncomfortable we might feel. Once we truly learn to reside in our fear of aloneness, we will no longer expect those we are intimate with to assume responsibility for taking away our fear or making us feel good. Instead we will know reality; we will know love.

The basic fear of aloneness may also include a related anxiety that is not usually recognized: the fear of disconnection—from others as well as from our own heart. This fear penetrates deeper than loneliness, and often manifests as a knotted quiver in the chest or abdomen. Remember, at bottom, the heart that seeks to awaken, to live genuinely, is more real than anything. It is the nameless drive that calls us to be who we most truly are. When we are not in touch with this, we may feel the existential anxiety of disconnection.

In a way, much of spiritual practice is geared toward helping us address our feeling of basic separation. How does this occur? First, we acknowledge our fear, and see it clearly for what it is. We need to remember that the fear is, in fact, our path itself, our direct route to experiencing the Being Kindness at our core.

Then we must face the fear directly, saying yes to it. Essentially, this means we are willing to experience it rather than run away from it. When fear arises, in order to replace our usual dread with a genuine curiosity, we might ask, "Here it is again, how will it be this time?" As we truly feel it, breathing the physical sensations of anxiety into the center of the chest, the familiar thoughts that normally fuel our fear begin to fall away, and we can experience the healing power of the heart. This is a nonconceptual experience—it does not come from words or explanations but rather from the spaciousness of a wider container of awareness. When the fear of living as a separate being dissolves, we naturally tap into the connectedness and Being Kindness that are always available to us, and that are the real fruit of the practice life.

Unworthiness

The third basic fear is that of unworthiness. This fear takes many forms, such as the fear that I don't count, the fear of general inadequacy, of being unworthy of love, of being nothing or stupid, and so on. The basic fear that we'll never measure up dictates much of our behavior; for example, for some, it impels us to continuously and forcefully prove ourselves, while for others, it might prompt us to cease trying. In either case, isn't our motivation the same: to avoid facing the basic fear of unworthiness? We may fear the feeling of unworthiness more than anything.

In fact, we are often merciless in these self-judgments of unworthiness—not just when we're upset at ourselves, but as an ongoing frame of mind. Even if they're not glaringly obvious, our self-judgments are always lurking under the surface, waiting to arise. For example, those who have stage fright, including the anxiety of public speaking, may feel the constant underground dread of having to deal with it. There's a joke that people can fear public speaking so intensely that at a funeral they would rather be in the casket than give the eulogy.

Fear of public speaking triggers the dread and shame of public failure and humiliation. But what is really being threatened? Isn't it just our self-image of appearing strong, calm, insightful, or whatever our own particular narrow view is of who we're supposed to be? We certainly fear appearing weak or not on top of it—why? Because that would confirm our own negative core beliefs of unworthiness. Even though there is no real danger, isn't it true that the fear of failing often *feels* fatal? Yet ironically, our very attempt to fight the fear is most often what increases it, and may even result in panic.

There is a better alternative: as with the other basic fears described in this chapter, to effectively work with the fear of unworthiness, we must learn to let it in willingly, to breathe the sensations of fear directly into the center of the chest. In other words, to say yes to the fear.

At one point in my life, when I was struggling with my fear of giving public talks, I joined Toastmasters, a group designed to help develop skills in public speaking. But I didn't join to learn to give better talks, or even with the goal of overcoming my fear. I joined so that I could have a laboratory, a place to invite the fear in and go to its roots. In a way, I actually began to look forward to the fear arising so that I could breathe it right into the heart, entering into it fully. Paradoxically, the willingness to be with the fear *completely* is what changes the experience of fear altogether. It's not that fear will no longer arise; it's that we no longer fear it.

Eventually, we all need to be willing to face the deepest, darkest beliefs we have about ourselves. Only in this way can we come to *know* that they are only beliefs, and not the truth about who we are. By willingly entering into this process, by seeing through the fiction of who we believe ourselves to be, we can connect with our true nature. As Nietzsche put it, "One must have chaos in oneself to give birth to a dancing star." Love is the dancing star, the fruit of saying yes, of consciously and willingly facing our fears.

When we can feel fear within the spaciousness of the breath and heart, we may even come to see it more as an adventure than a nightmare. To see it as an adventure means being willing to take the ride with curiosity, even with its inevitable ups and downs. Over the years, because I've had to speak in public quite frequently, this situation has provided an opportunity to tap into what is really important to me: to remember that my aspiration is to learn to live from Being Kindness. Whenever I've remembered this right before giving a talk, it was no longer an issue of whether or not I felt the discomfort of anxiety. This allowed me to say yes to it, and to willingly breathe the anxiety right in. In other words, when we connect with a larger sense of what life is, negative core beliefs such as "I'll never measure up" may still come up, but they no longer dictate how we feel and live. Instead, we begin to use the fear as our actual path to learning to live from Being Kindness.

Remember, it's a given that we don't want to feel the fear of unworthiness, but at some point we have to understand that it's more painful to try to suppress our fears and self-judgments, thus solidifying them, than it is to actually feel them. This is part of what it means to bring Being Kindness to our practice, because we are no longer viewing our fear as proof that we're defective. Without Being Kindness, regardless of how much discipline we have, regardless of how serious we are about practice, we will still stay stuck in the subtle mercilessness of the mind, telling us we are basically and fundamentally unworthy. We should never underestimate the need for Being Kindness on the long and sometimes daunting path of learning to awaken.

Please note that these three basic fears— insecurity and helplessness, aloneness and disconnection, and unworthiness—are not just mental. Scientists tell us that fear is written into the cellular memory of the body, particularly into a small part of the brain called the amygdala. That is why simply knowing about our fears intellectually will not free us from their domination. Every time they are triggered, we slide into an established groove in the brain. Nonetheless, we still have to see our fears clearly before we can practice with them directly.

When I was a child, my father told me repeatedly, "The only thing to fear is fear itself." Although his intentions were good, what I actually heard was that I should be afraid of fear! Fear thus became the enemy. We have to remember that fear is neither an enemy nor an obstacle; it is not a real monster. When we feel fear, we need to remind ourselves that it is our path; and when we truly understand this, we can actually welcome the physical experience of fear into the spaciousness of the heart.

Interestingly, it is this nonconceptual experiencing of our fears that allows the grooves in the brain, which are preprogrammed to react to fear, to slowly be filled in. How this works is a mystery. Not a mystery, however, is the fact that unless we can clearly see our individual fears for what they are, it is unlikely we will overcome our habitual and instinctive aversions to them. Conversely, once we are able to face our fears, we are one major step closer to living from Being Kindness. When we really let fear in, it is a portal to reality.

It is imperative that we return again and again to what is most real. I recently read about a financial advisor who didn't ask about his clients' specific financial goals; instead, he would ask them what they would do with their lives if they had just one week to live. Invariably the answers had to do with their real priorities, such as the wish to give back or to connect. The advisor would then tell them to let their financial goals reflect these real priorities, so that their lives wouldn't be dictated just by their fear and their needs for security and safety. Likewise for us, we can ask what would we want to do if we had just one week to live. If we can get in touch with what's really important, we can then begin to turn away, little by little, from our fear-based behaviors that keep us locked in a self-imposed exile. Only then can we truly live from the love that is our essential nature.

14

Relationships and Love

"WHAT IS HELL? Hell is the suffering of being unable to love," wrote Dostoevsky in *The Brothers Karamazov*. Indeed, we may have knowledge and deep insight, but without Being Kindness, something essential will always be lacking. Until we can truly surrender to love, our aspiration to live most genuinely will not be fulfilled.

What is love? Love is actually very difficult to discuss because it means so many different things to different people—from sexual love, to romantic love, to friendship love, to family love, and so on. The one thing these various kinds of love have in common is that they are all forms of personal love, where we are so often caught up in the highs and lows of emotion and attachment. But there is another kind of love, one that is not even an emotion—it is the natural state of our being. This love is what naturally comes forth when all the conditions that we add to our relationships—our agendas, our needs, our expectations—stop getting in the way.

Yet, isn't it true that we rarely experience this sort of love? Isn't it much more common to experience relationships as a source of difficulty? I'm not just talking about relationships with our mates, but also with our parents, our children, our bosses, our friends, and even with strangers we interact with at random throughout the day. So why is there so much difficulty? Or, more pointedly, what is it that each of us brings to relationships that seems to cause so many problems?

The answer is: ourselves! We bring our assumptions, our hopes, and most of all, our wants. Whenever we want something from someone, which is always true when we have expectations and requirements of them, we can't really see them as people. We only see them in terms of what we want them to provide. And as long as we want something from them, our capacity for love is blocked. This might lead to difficulties around intimacy or trust, around fears of criticism or rejection, or around feeling unappreciated or controlled. Certainly money issues and sexual issues can cause us difficulties.

Given these inevitable difficulties, relationships often test us, pushing us to the edges of where we're stuck. But even though being pushed in this way is uncomfortable, it affords us the invaluable opportunity to go deeper into our life, and to reconnect with the unconditional love that is our true nature. We may think that the difficulties of a relationship will prevent or distract us from our desired journey on the spiritual path; we may think that in order to know ourselves more deeply, we have to ascend the mountaintop alone. But the issues that arise in relationships can, in fact, push us in ways that we would never push ourselves on our own, in spite of the sincerity of our quest. And it's this very fact, that relationships often trigger our most painful and unhealed emotions, that makes them such a potentially useful teacher.

There are three main steps essential to working with relationships—knowing oneself, refraining and experiencing, and practicing Being Kindness. Taken together, these three steps will help us learn to live from our true nature.

Knowing Oneself

To see clearly what you really want from a relationship, or at least what you believe you want, think of one important relationship where you've experienced difficulties. Now consider the following questions: What is this relationship supposed to give me? What are my specific expectations of this person?

We often want other people to be a certain way, primarily so that we'll feel a certain way, such as safe, confident, loved, pleasured, happy, appreciated, and so forth. For example, when we believe someone loves us and wants us, we not only feel loved but also worthy of love, which is often the balm we crave to cover over our basic fears of unworthiness. But if our needs and expectations are not met in that relationship, we often feel unloved, rejected, lonely, and unappreciated. Again, think of your own situation to see how this specifically applies. We need to see that almost all of our relationship difficulties come from our wanting someone or something to be different.

Often compounding or intensifying relationship difficulties is the fact that we almost always enter into relations unaware of our expectations. I met my first wife in a spiritual community, and thought at the time that I wanted nothing more than a partner on my spiritual journey. But what I also unknowingly wanted was someone to pay attention to me and appreciate me, and this lack of awareness eventually caused unending difficulties.

The point is, one of the most basic aspects of practicing with relationships is to become clear about our own specific expectations and agendas. We need to know, very precisely, both how we want another to be and how we want them to make us feel. The more clearly we see our assumptions and patterns, the more our unrealistic and self-defeating views of relationship will be slowly dismantled. The surrender of our illusions—about what relationship is, and particularly about what it's supposed to do for me—is essential. But in order to surrender, we first have to learn to see ourselves more clearly.

Again, thinking of your own particular situation, when you don't get what you want, or when you get what you don't want—that is, when your expectations aren't met—what are your typical emotional reactions? Are you prone to anger, hurt, self-pity, anxiety, depression, fear? It's important to be clear about what your particular emotional reactions are; otherwise, relationships will remain a mystery, and their difficulties may seem to be unworkable.

We tend to view relationship difficulties as obstacles, as impediments to our happiness, and sometimes even to our spiritual path. Usually, when these difficulties arise and we get upset, we automatically believe that something is wrong. Then we jump to the belief "I have to fix this." But in doing so, we're missing a crucial point, which is seeing that these obstacles, these difficulties, can themselves be a step on the path of awakening. They are not in our way so much as they *are* our way.

We often forget that difficulties present the most valuable opportunities to learn about ourselves, especially about our own barriers. In relationships, the other person is, in fact, a mirror reflecting back to us exactly what needs clarifying—our expectations, our judgments, our anger, and our fear. In this sense, rather than seeing the other person as the cause of our suffering, we begin to see that person as our teacher, indirectly pointing to what we must attend to in order to live from Being Kindness.

This is an important point—we don't have to travel far to find a relationship guru; our guru is the very person who pushes our buttons, who shows us all the ways in which we are stuck, all the places where our patterns, attitudes, and actions block our way to Being Kindness. This is one of the beauties of relationship as spiritual practice.

But even just remembering to see our relationship difficulties within the context of practice is a big, and often incredibly difficult, step. How often do we view our difficulties in this way? For example, if someone is critical toward us, or betrays us, how often do we remember that they're our teacher? Yet, when we don't remember this, aren't we perpetuating our own cycle of suffering, and the hurting of ourselves and others?

When difficulties arise, we must first remember that this is about us, and that our struggle is our opportunity to wake up to exactly what we need to work with. For example, as we hear thoughts such as "I can't stand it when he does that," "Nobody should be treated this way," "This just isn't right," or "Why does she always do that?" can we begin to see them as clues that practice is necessary. This means to see them clearly as just deeply believed thoughts coming out of us, out of our conditioning. It's important to understand that our thoughts, no matter how strong, are not necessarily The Truth. And even if they sound objectively "right," we can ask ourselves whether they in fact foster righteousness rather than relatedness.

Refraining and Experiencing

As a result of our emotional reactions in relationships, we often engage in power struggles, trying to change others to suit us, or withholding something they want until they give us what we want. Think of a difficult relationship. Can you see how you're often unwilling to give, primarily because you're not getting what you want, and how quickly a power struggle ensues before you're even aware of its roots?

In relationships, particularly when we have an emotional reaction, we'll almost always focus on the other person instead of looking inward. What we're really trying to do is change that person so they'll fulfill our hopes and expectations. In these power struggles, we may even view the other person as our enemy, which leads us to either erect barriers of protection or attack in order to defend ourselves. We must be honest about this.

Even when we intellectually know that our emotional upset is the result of bringing our own expectations and agendas to the situation, it is often difficult to see this clearly when we're upset. And even when we do see it, it's still difficult to work with. Why? *Because it means that we have to stop blaming others.* This point is crucial. Whenever we find ourselves wanting to point the blaming finger at someone or something outside of ourselves, we can gradually learn to turn the finger around and look at what we ourselves are doing. This does not mean that we blame ourselves; it means that we stop blaming altogether.

The problem is, we don't want to stop blaming. It is one of our choice detours away from reality. We often *want* to be angry, to be right. We like the juiciness and power that we feel when we're angry. But in order to work with relationship difficulties, we have to recognize the tenacity of these defensive strategies of blaming and righteousness. And here's where it gets really sticky, because once we do stop holding on to blame and defense, we are left with the one thing that we least want to experience—the quivering core of fear that we have tried all of our lives to avoid. We have to realize that the reason we focus on blaming someone else is to cover over having to feel this fear-based pain. We don't want to feel the discomfort of that.

The practice emphasis is to come back again and again to our own inner process; yet, it's important to note that sometimes we may encounter situations that objectively require action, sometimes even right away. But whenever possible, it's best to clarify our interior landscape before taking action, since it is likely that unless we have first worked with our own negativity, we will make matters worse.

As an example of the predictable pattern of blame, let's say a difficulty arises as the result of feeling criticized. We may immediately feel hurt, which is almost always based in fear. All of the old memories of hurt may come rising out of the cellar, and it's quite possible that the strength of our emotional reaction is based more on the accumulation of past hurts than on the current situation. The beliefs that stem from these accumulated hurts go screaming through our head: "This always happens to me!" "How could she treat me like that?" "See, I knew nobody could be trusted," "I'm so stupid!" or "I can't take this." And we certainly believe these thoughts to be true, especially when we're right in the middle of our reaction. Since it's painful to experience them, we move immediately into avoidance, into our own particular defensive strategy, such as blaming, withdrawing, or seeking diversions.

Whatever our particular defensive pattern is, we have to see that this behavior or strategy, while arising as a means of avoiding feeling the painful quality of our emotional reaction, is not the same as the emotion itself. Furthermore, the only way to actually *feel* the emotion—to say yes to it, to work with and heal it—is to first refrain from the defensive behavioral strategy. Only by refraining from our defensive strategies, particularly the pattern of blaming, can we stay in the present moment of our emotional reactions.

Residing in our emotional reactions most often leads us to the very uncomfortable feeling of fear, which can be the hardest thing of all to stay with. But can you see how fear is a key issue underlying most of our relationship difficulties? Fear, more than anything, is what blocks intimacy and love. These fears may not be immediately apparent, but they're there nonetheless. And they continue to exert a powerful, even overpowering, influence until they're addressed.

But what, exactly, do we fear? Think of your own situation. Can you identify your own particular core fears? Can you see the extent to which these fears drive you, even if you're not feeling them now? In order to practice with difficulties in relationships, it's important to first understand the specific dynamic fear takes within yourself. Some examples include the fears of being abandoned or rejected, of not getting what we want or losing what we have, of intimacy, of being overwhelmed, of losing control or being controlled, of feeling unloved or unworthy, and so on.

These fears are not necessarily logical or reasonable. For example, fearing that we're unworthy of love doesn't mean it's true. It just means that we believe it to be true; consequently, so long as we remain caught in our belief, that fear will control the way we act, react, and relate to others. So first, we have to begin to see clearly our own particular fears, since they underlie almost all of our relationship conflicts.

Then comes the most difficult part of practicing with relationship difficulties—where we have to be willing to be present with, to really *feel* this core quiver of fear-based pain. Knowing our thoughts is important, but this in itself cannot touch our accumulated memory of pain. It's so easy to stay mired in blame, replaying old wounds, but we may eventually find that it's not necessary to stay stuck on the history channel; it's always possible to switch to the discovery channel, where we begin to look at our experience in a new way. The task itself is very straightforward, yet it is nonetheless very difficult to do: we need to refrain from replaying our story line of drama and blame and instead say yes to the present moment of our experience—to actually feel it, to rest in the bodily sensations no matter how uncomfortable they may be. We might think we can't stand it, but of course we can. We just don't want to.

One practice technique mentioned earlier—the Three Breaths Practice—may help when the pain seems too much to bear. Again, we simply tell the ego, which is the source of resistance, that we will only feel the painful feelings for the duration of three breaths. After that, we'll divert ourselves into fantasy or another source of comfort—whatever our form of "chocolate" may be. Then we feel the emotion—that most dreaded thing we haven't wanted to feel—fully and with intention for three breaths. After that, we don't renege on the deal; we allow ourselves to turn away. We do, however, come back to experiencing again and again later, three breaths at a time.

Awareness is what heals. This is the most basic principle of spiritual practice. Awareness is what makes our suffering less solid. As we begin to see through our fears, as they become more porous, they no longer run our behavior, they no longer cause so much pain.

Until we face our fears, we will not be able to truly connect with others, because we'll still be disconnected from ourselves. If we don't become intimate with our own fears, how can we have a healthy relationship with another who is also caught in fear? But as we learn to befriend our fears, we no longer fear them; and when we meet someone who may be angry at us, instead of immediately reacting to the anger, we may understand that they're really just afraid. The path to awakening the heart of compassion toward another is always rooted in our acceptance of our own pain.

Once we become familiar with our own fears, we may find it helpful to communicate them to those who are closest to us. I remember sitting in a restaurant with Elizabeth in the first months of our relationship. It was right before a retreat, and for whatever reason, my Pandora's box of fears was wide open. I had never before spoken openly to another person in a detailed way about my fears, mostly out of shame, not wanting to appear weak. But in the prior months of learning to say yes to feeling my fears, I no longer saw them as my enemy nor as defeat; so that evening, I chose to tell Elizabeth how I was feeling without holding anything back.

What amazed me was that she simply listened without comment or judgment. It's rare to feel heard, to feel met with Being Kindness, but it's particularly satisfying when we are feeling exposed. The risk we take is being misunderstood, judged, or rejected; but it's worth the risk if our aspiration is to truly connect with another. Honestly sharing our fears is an essential step toward true intimacy in relationships. But in order to do this, we must first be willing to welcome the difficulties that inevitably arise.

This may sound like a somewhat dark and perhaps even bleak view of relationships. You may wish to forget this seemingly grim talk about saying yes to our pain and our fears. You may prefer to focus on the more positive aspects of relationships, or think that if something feels bad, the relationship is not healthy. As human beings, we naturally want to lighten up and focus on finding pleasure or comfort in our relationships; but we have to understand that as long as there is suffering in our relationships, we need to bring attention to those areas where we are most stuck.

Through this work, we can come to know the real meaning of love in relationship, no longer settling for superficial security or the comfort of psychological safety. The more we defuse the conditions that we ourselves have imposed on our relationships—the judgments, the perceived wants and needs—the more the path is cleared for love to simply flow through us. Of course, some things will yield more gracefully than others, and we shouldn't be glib about the tremendous challenges we face here.

Practicing Being Kindness

There's an additional step we can take in our work with relationships: practicing Being Kindness toward those we are having difficulty with as well as toward ourselves. We can certainly do this during the Being Kindness meditation, but we can also do it in our outward behavior, through intentional acts of giving in daily life.

This is, however, a very tricky area, because trying to act from kindness can easily become a moral dictate that bypasses the pain we feel deep inside. For example, if someone is mean to us and we feel hurt, it would not be helpful to try to act kindly in return without *also* addressing what's really going on inside of us. Such kindness would be more cosmetic than real; it's possibly a way to hold on to the image we want to have of ourselves as a kind person. By trying to change our behavior to fit into a more ideal version of ourselves, we are right back in the world of Me-stuff. Besides, this type of effort is eventually bound to backfire, because it bypasses the anger and fear underneath that prevent us from giving genuine kindness in the first place.

Conversely, when we're willing to acknowledge our own interior and often rocky landscape, making intentional acts of kindness can be very fruitful, in that they allow us to face within ourselves whatever discomfort arises from these actions. This is particularly true when we realize that the most difficult thing for us to give to another is often what the other wants most. Think of someone close to you. What does this person want most from you that you're unwilling to give? I'm talking about something you're capable of giving, but hold back on out of fear, either a conscious fear or one of which you're not even aware. Take a minute to consider this.

Here's an example: if what our partner wants most from us is acceptance, to act intentionally from kindness would mean that we refrain from criticizing and stop trying to make that person be different from who he or she is. This may sound impossible, or at least very difficult, but consider what's at stake. If we could honestly give nonjudgment to another as an act of kindness, it would force us to work with exactly what we most need to work with—our own fears and attachments around our judgments. Besides, consider how much it might mean to the other to be met with kindness.

We may encounter strong resistance when giving to another what the other wants, particularly if we have been keeping track of grievances for a long time. Still, as we work through the layers of anger, fear, and discomfort underlying our resistance, we'll be freeing ourselves from our own inner barriers. We ordinarily believe that the barriers to love lie in the other person, but these barriers are always our own.

Although we usually assume another person can and should be able to take away our discomfort, this assumption is a major obstruction to experiencing genuine connectedness and love. From a practice point of view, working with discomfort is primarily our own inner work. Because the practice of giving to another will no doubt highlight our discomfort, doing so allows us to intentionally work with our own pain and fear that are at the root of that discomfort. The practice of giving in this way can thus be our exact path to living from the Being Kindness that is our true nature.

A student told me about how she really didn't want to go on a trip her husband wanted to go on, but decided to intentionally work with her own fears by giving him what he wanted. Although she didn't mention it to him, this meant dealing with her beliefs that what she wanted didn't matter, and the consequent fear of being discounted. The trip got planned, but a few days before they were going to leave, he told her that they had to cancel. When she heard this, she burst into tears, thinking how disappointed he must have been. He then confessed that the only reason he planned the trip was because he thought she wanted to go! They got a good laugh out of that, but the important thing is that she made the intentional effort to give him what she thought he wanted, as a means of working with her deepest fears. Once she had worked with this, there was no residual resentment, as evidenced by her tears at what she imagined was his disappointment. What started as an intentional effort was transformed into a genuine act of giving from kindness.

The point is, we don't have to try to feel loving or kind; we just have to work with what gets in the way, particularly where we hold our hearts back in fear. Interestingly, once we work with our own fears, others will often feel the freedom to move toward us. And when others no longer feel the need to defend, they too may become more willing to work with their own stuck places, and we, in turn, will feel more freedom to move toward them.

None of this is guaranteed, of course; but at least it opens the door to a place where two people can learn to truly connect, without defense. Undefended, it's the nature of the heart to give; and love on this level is the natural wanting to do things for another without needing anything in return. But remember, relating to another in this way can be very difficult, especially when we're in the midst of our own upsets. This is why perseverance, coupled with the ability to extend Being Kindness toward ourselves, is so crucial. This gives us the courage not to give up on ourselves, and in turn not to give up on others. As we stop holding ourselves back in fear and learn to give from the heart, it's increasingly possible to find the love in relationship that we all seek. This doesn't mean we won't have preferences about our loved one's behavior; but there's an enormous difference between having a preference and placing an emotional demand on the other person.

In actively practicing Being Kindness through intentional acts of giving, we may even come to understand the deeper meaning of the biblical phrase "love thy neighbor as thyself." This is often seen as a moral dictate, an injunction to change our behavior. But on a deeper level, it can be seen as a statement about the nature of reality. Very specifically, when we truly experience our basic connectedness, and tap into the Being Kindness that is our essential nature, we automatically love others *as ourselves* because we no longer see ourselves as separate from others. This understanding may only come intermittently, and perhaps only in brief glimpses, but we can't lose sight of its fundamental truth.

The alternative is to continue to live stuck in fear. When we live from fear, relating to others as separate from us, we consequently see them as a threat. But when we no longer run away from our own fear and suffering—instead experiencing them fully by breathing them directly into the heart—we are able to see the suffering of others as no different from our own. Opening up in this way to the universal suffering of humanity allows us to see others as they really are, free from the filters of our own needs and fears. This brings us closer to fulfilling our life task: to know the truth of who we really are—that the nature of our being is connectedness and love. This is what it means to live from the Zen Heart. Our task is not to change ourselves or others, but to know the world through love. Through our conscious suffering we can connect with the broader pain of humanity; and through the breath into the center of the chest we enter into the spacious heart of connectedness.

As we begin to know the world through love, our actions in the world come more and more naturally from a true understanding of who we are. And when situations arise where we don't know what to do or say, we can ask the pivotal practice question, "What would it mean, in this very moment, to live from Being Kindness?" As we breathe into the center of the chest, we allow the answer to come not from the mind but from the heart.

It is at this point that our personal love begins to merge with the bigger love that is our true nature. Our personal love becomes a portal to Big Love and also a channel through which Big Love can flow. For example, when I experience Big Love, I immediately think of Elizabeth, who becomes the channel through which that love is directed. As well, sometimes when I look at Elizabeth and see her kind heart and deep aspiration, I naturally step through the portal into Big Love. The love is then directed toward all equally, the same way the sun shines on everything without discrimination. Being Kindness is devoid of judgment; it excludes no one. It embraces all and everything. Love gives without the expectation that it will get something in return. Love gives with no agenda, with no purpose. Love, on this level, simply is. It is the natural state of our unobstructed being.

15
Three Heart Meditations

THE THIRD ESSENTIAL PHASE in spiritual practice involves learning to actually live from Being Kindness. Three specific meditation practices—the Being Kindness Meditation, the Heart of Compassion Meditation, and the Healing Meditation—although only a part of this phase of practice, have been found by many to be very powerful learning tools.

So what, exactly, is Being Kindness? We could define Being Kindness as a sense of connectedness, of innate goodwill, perhaps accompanied by receptivity and warmth. There is a sense of openness that diminishes the mind's tendency to constantly judge. In fact, the practices of Being Kindness cultivate unconditional friendliness, because we no longer push away aspects of ourselves as unwanted or bad.

Traditional loving-kindness practice, often referred to as *metta* practice, has a similar orientation. Metta is about cultivating an attitude of mind in which we desire the welfare of everyone, including ourselves. The essence of the traditional loving-kindness meditation is the repetition of certain phrases, such as "May I be happy" and "May all beings be happy." The point is to generate the feeling of loving-kindness or boundless love. The three meditations presented here are also a means of cultivating a compassionate attitude of mind, which is an essential part of the Buddhist tradition.

However, the three meditations in this chapter have a somewhat different orientation, in that they don't focus on trying

to make us feel a particular way, but rather on bringing awareness to what we are feeling right in this moment, including our
anger and fear. The loving-kindness meditation as it is often
presented bypasses dealing directly with our anger and fear,
but if the practice stops with saying affirmations such as "May
I be happy" or "May I be peaceful," it is easy to detour away
from a genuine Being Kindness practice and instead generate
a superficial loving or kind feeling. The latter merely covers over
the pain we need to bring into awareness. Here, rather than trying to seem more "loving," we'll start with the basic understanding that at the deepest level, the heart of Being Kindness is
who we are; it is the nature of our being. Thus, practicing with
these three meditations becomes a means by which we learn to
awaken the heart.

The meditation practices presented here also differ from
traditional metta practices in that the focus is not so much on
mental phrases, such as "May I be happy," as it is on the physical experience of breathing into the center of the chest. Staying
with awareness of the breath into the area of the heart not only
keeps us based in physical reality but also paradoxically under-
cuts the forcefulness and solidity of the judgmental mind. This
allows us to access our natural capacity to be open, to relate
with a heartfelt friendliness to ourselves and to others, exactly
as we are.

However, it can't be emphasized enough that we are not
using these Heart meditations to generate a good feeling. Rather,
we are attending to how we are right now. Interestingly, this will
often include attending to whatever keeps our natural kindness
from coming forth. For example, we may contact the anger
and fear that are usually underneath our unkindness. In fact, as
these unwanted qualities are encountered with nonjudgmental
awareness, it's less likely that they will burst forth in unskillful
words and actions. Instead, acknowledging and experiencing

the anger and fear may allow our natural kindness to gradually begin to flow.

The Being Kindness Meditation

This meditation, which is an offshoot of the traditional loving-kindness meditation, consists of three-line rounds that repeat several times. The first round is oriented toward oneself; the second and following rounds are directed toward people close to you; the last round includes everyone.

The three lines of this meditation correspond to the three basic stages of practice described in this book. The first line, "attending to what blocks the path," corresponds to the work done in the Me Phase of practice—the long and difficult stage of working with all of our protections, fears, and judgments. The second line, "being aware in this moment, just as it is," corresponds to the phase of Being Awareness, where we settle into a larger sense of what life is. The last line, "extending Being Kindness to everyone," corresponds to the phase of Being Kindness, where we learn to live from the awakened heart.

Understanding the lines of this meditation within the context of the three phases of practice allows us to use them to continuously connect to the bigger picture. The actual words and lines of the Being Kindness Meditation are also important in that they help us to focus and direct our attention. Naturally, as in any other meditation, we will tend to wander off into daydreams, plans, and fantasies. But in staying with the words and lines as best we can, we'll at the very least sharpen our focus.

I consider the following meditation to be one of the single most important and powerful practices I've encountered. However, please note that it is not meant to replace daily sitting, but rather to complement it. If it is not possible to do the Being

Kindness Meditation at a separate time, it can be included at the end of your regular sitting.

Finally, if you already do a loving-kindness meditation, try setting it aside for a while and try this meditation instead, so that you can be more open to whatever may be of value here.

To begin the Being Kindness Meditation, take a couple of deep breaths. Become aware of the breath and begin to follow it into the center of the chest. Experience the area around the heart. Does it feel closed and constricted? Does it feel clear and open? Does it feel warm or cool? Is it neutral? Whatever you feel, just be aware of that. With each in-breath, breathe as if the breath is being pulled directly into the center of the chest. With each in-breath, let awareness go a little deeper.

Then, as a warm-up, to help activate your innate Being Kindness, silently say the three opening lines in conjunction with your breathing.

The first part of each line, "*Breathing into the heart,*" should be said on the in-breath. As you breathe in, feel the experience of dwelling in the heart. The second and remaining part of each line should then be said on the out-breath.

Stay with each line for two to three breaths, so that the words can be translated into a bodily experience.

> "Breathing into the heart, no one to be."
> "Breathing into the heart, nothing to do."
> "Breathing into the heart, just Being."

Allow yourself to dwell in the heart. Allow any warmth that may be present in the heart region to extend on the out-breath to your whole body, your whole being. If there is no warmth, no Being Kindness to extend, simply notice this, or whatever else may be present, and continue.

First Round: To Yourself

The first round of this meditation is directed toward yourself. Again, the first part of each line, "*Breathing into the heart,*" is said silently on the in-breath, while the second part is said silently on the out-breath. It is best to stay with each line for a few breaths before going on to the next one.

The first line:

> "Breathing into the heart, attending to what blocks Being Kindness."

Become aware of any aspect of yourself—anger, self-protections, self-judgment—that blocks access to the open heart. You can also become aware of any contraction or tension anywhere in the body. Extend the warmth and Being Kindness of awareness into these aspects of yourself, *wherever you can feel them.* Remember, you are not trying to get rid of anything. Rather, you are extending the compassion of awareness to these very closed-off areas, as an act of Being Kindness.

The second line:

> "Breathing into the heart, being aware in this moment, just as it is."

Become aware of everything around and within you— sounds, smells, sights, physical sensations, mood, thoughts— and let yourself experience a larger sense of what life is; let everything be just as it is. This experience is very similar to the Three Point Awareness Meditation, where we are simultaneously aware of the breath into the center of the chest, the spaciousness of the environment, and the overall sense, or gestalt, of the body—the sense that "I am here." When the mind wanders, softly come back to the awareness of breath and heart, without self-judgment.

The third line:

> "Breathing into the heart, extending Being Kindness to everyone."

Extend whatever Being Kindness arises to other beings, including any specific people who may come into your awareness.

Repeat the following three lines to yourself:

> "Breathing into the heart, attending to what blocks Being Kindness."
> "Breathing into the heart, being aware in this moment, just as it is."
> "Breathing into the heart, extending Being Kindness to everyone."

Repeat the three lines to yourself one more time.

Second Round: To Others

Now bring into awareness the presence of someone close to you, for whom you have positive feelings, to whom you wish to extend Being Kindness.

Breathe the person's image, her presence, into the center of the chest on the in-breath. On the out-breath, extend Being Kindness toward this person while repeating the three lines. If you feel resistance, just acknowledge it and experience whatever is in the way. Stay with each line for the duration of a few breaths.

> "Breathing (name) into the heart, may she be healed in her difficulties."
> "Breathing (name) into the heart, may she be aware in this moment, just as it is."
> "Breathing (name) into the heart, may she extend Being Kindness to everyone."

Choose another person for whom you have positive feelings and repeat the three lines again, remembering to breathe in and out of the center of the chest as you say the words of Being Kindness.

Choose one more person, perhaps someone with whom you are having difficulty, and repeat the three lines again. Don't be surprised if there is resistance. Just notice and feel its physical texture while continuing to stay in touch with breath and heart.

If you would like to include more people, take a few breaths between each round. Always remember to stay physically grounded by keeping awareness on the breath and the center of the chest.

Third Round: To Everyone

Finally, expand the main focus to all beings. Bring awareness into the center of the chest on the in-breath, repeating the first part of each line; and with the out-breath, repeat the remainder of each line, allowing Being Kindness to be extended to everyone.

> "Breathing everyone into the heart, may they be healed in their difficulties."
> "Breathing everyone into the heart, may they be aware in this moment, just as it is."

"Breathing everyone into the heart, may they extend Being Kindness to one another."

Ending

After completing all three rounds, come back to simply breathing in and out of the center of the chest, experiencing the texture and quality of the heart. Dwelling in the heart, go deeper with each in-breath as you repeat the three lines that began the meditation:

"Breathing into the heart, no one to be."
"Breathing into the heart, nothing to do."
"Breathing into the heart, just Being."

NOTES ON THE BEING KINDNESS MEDITATION

In order to experience the power of this practice, it is important to do the Being Kindness Meditation regularly. Doing it for a long period of time, such as for a whole day at a retreat, is also very instructive.

If you find the particular words of the Being Kindness Meditation awkward, you can experiment with changing them so that they are more meaningful to you.

Sometimes students ask if these lines are the same as affirmations. The answer is no. Affirmations are often a mental exercise that is used to change our feelings or circumstances. The lines of the Being Kindness Meditation are not about changing anything; they're about experiencing whatever is present within the spaciousness of the heart.

Furthermore, the Being Kindness practice is not a mental exercise; its focus is on *physical awareness* in the center of the chest. All of the images, all of the lines, are experienced through awareness of the breath in and out of this area. So the words are invitations to what is already inherent to come forth, rather than an attempt to change ourselves or our situation.

When first doing this meditation, it may feel uncomfortable to experience the breath in and out of the center of the chest. It may also feel foreign to silently repeat the words of Being Kindness. But even if you experience discomfort or cynicism, it's worth the effort to stay with this practice. I know of no other practice so effective in undercutting the perniciousness of the judgmental mind or in helping break through our chronic state of separateness. Breathing in and out of the center of the chest has a power that can't be explained or denied; and the only way to experience this power is to make the Being Kindness Meditation a regular part of your practice life.

Some people find the openness of the Being Kindness Meditation threatening, so don't be surprised if doing this practice brings up doubt and resistance, or even contempt. It is also common to feel that you are deceiving yourself—that the experience of Being Kindness may not be genuine. But even if you believe these negative thoughts, it doesn't mean that they're true. The more you can avoid getting caught in your judgmental mind, the more you can be open to what's of value.

As we practice Being Kindness on a regular basis, it is no longer just a meditation exercise. It becomes a part of our being, our natural response to life. And whenever we feel stuck, we can ask the pivotal question, "In this very moment, what would it mean to live from Being Kindness?"

We may discover that when fear arises, we can see it, experience it, and learn to send nonjudgmental awareness into this fearful being. When illness arises, instead of seeing ourselves as defective or analyzing how we are ill because of this or that, we can breathe into the heart, experiencing the "whatness" of who we are in that moment. We then extend Being Kindness into our physical body. This practice teaches us that we can receive even the most unwanted aspects of ourselves with a certain sense of unconditional friendliness, a quality that captures the essence of an awakened heart.

The Heart of Compassion Meditation

Sometimes, when we feel overwhelmed, nothing we've learned about practice seems helpful. In this dark place, where we feel hopeless, helpless, and out of control, we become so deeply caught in our own drama that we can't even imagine a way out. During such times, the following meditation may be particularly helpful. The purpose of this meditation is to move out of the very narrow focus on ourselves, so that we can connect with the healing experience of tapping into the pain of others. At first glance, this may sound like a morose endeavor, but paradoxically, awareness of the suffering of others is the exact antidote to our self-absorbed sense of hopelessness. Suffering is often the most effective vehicle for awakening the heart.

To begin the Heart of Compassion Meditation, first sit for a while, bringing attention to the center of the chest via the breath. Feel the texture, the quality, in the heart area.

Bring to mind your own physical or emotional distress. Feel it, as physically as possible, rather than focusing on the story line.

Then bring to mind people who have the same or similar difficulties you are dealing with, such as illness, fear, shame, and so on. You can imagine the many people all over the world who share this pain; and as you think of them, breathe this image into the heart on the in-breath. And, on the out-breath, extend to them your wish that they be healed in their difficulties.

Feel the universality of the pain all people share. You are not taking on the burden of other people's pain; you are only bringing awareness to the fact that many people are suffering as you are.

Then again feel your own pain. On the in-breath, breathe the sensations of yourself in pain into the center of the chest, and on the out-breath, extend to yourself the wish to be healed.

As you stay with your distress, feel the sense of kinship with all of the other people who share in this pain. Feel the universality of the "shared being," the sense of connectedness with all people and life. This is the heartfelt sense of kinship with humanity. This is the awakened heart that can encompass pain with compassion.

Continue breathing in your distress, extending a benign awareness toward yourself, connecting with the shared pain and the shared being of humanity.

Even if you don't connect with the shared pain or the shared being, just come back to simply breathing in and out of the center of the chest for a few minutes. Feel the texture there. Rest in the spaciousness of the heart.

Two-Line Version

Here is a two-line version of the above meditation that can be used instantly any time you are caught in a strong fear: First, think of a friend who has a similar fear, and extend Being Kindness to this person by breathing him or her into the center of the chest on the in-breath. On the out-breath, say the line, "May you be healed in your difficulty."

Then, on the very next in-breath, breathe the sensations of your own fear into the center of the chest, and on the out-breath, extend Being Kindness to yourself in the same way you did toward the friend.

For some reason, when we tap into the innate desire to wish another well, we can more easily channel that wish for well-being toward ourselves.

The Healing Meditation

It is very unlikely that we can avoid the experience of physical pain or illness. Sometimes, pain comes on suddenly and can be acute. Other times, we may have to deal with prolonged or even chronic discomfort. In either case, it is helpful to have a healing meditation that can help us directly.

I have worked with this particular meditation for over twenty years, since I first began my adventure with a chronic illness of the immune system, whose main symptoms are nausea and weakness. The essence of the meditation is to stay present with the physical symptoms while directing the breath from the heart to the physical distress. Often, I find some degree of physical relief. In fact, sometimes the experience of nausea will transform into a more neutral physical energy.

I'm always astounded by the degree of equanimity and appreciation that can result from this meditation. But of course such results are not guaranteed; just as often, discomfort remains. However, at the very least, by doing the meditation I've entered more deeply into the heart.

My own practice in this area has shown me that healing (not cure) comes from simply staying with the "what" of my experiences. Many people try to find healing by looking for psychological explanations for their illness, but healing comes not from looking for explanations, nor from solely digging into our psychology or our past; healing comes from staying with the "whatness" of the moment, with all of the feelings and thoughts that need to be addressed—our fear, anger, shame, self-pity, and so on. As these feelings arise, we learn to stay with the experience while continuing to breathe in and out of the center of the chest. This is how we begin to heal in the bigger sense, connecting with a more spacious sense of what life is. This is how even illness and physical pain become our path.

As far as what cures what, who can say? Article after article touts their ninety-plus percent cure rates; yet, illness proliferates. I can feel within myself the *wanting* to believe that something might make me symptom-free—the wanting that stems from our deep-seated aversion to the fear of helplessness and loss of control. But using the Healing Meditation, I come back again and again to simply asking, "What is this moment?" and then residing in whatever arises.

One of the greatest gifts of my symptoms over the years has been the opportunity to work with the layers and layers of deeply-held believed thoughts and constricting emotions. This has enabled me to see through what prevents real healing—healing not based on physical comfort but on the awakening of the heart.

Instructions for the Healing Meditation

Take a few deep breaths in order to bring awareness into the body. Feel the place, or places, where discomfort is strongest. Then begin breathing into the center of the chest on the in-breath, and extending awareness to the places of discomfort (one at a time) on the out-breath.

It may be helpful to lightly place the fingers of one hand on the center of the chest, and the fingers of the other hand on the place of discomfort.

Continue breathing into the heart on the in-breath, and extending the wish to heal on the out-breath.

It is important that you don't view discomfort as your enemy, as something to get rid of. Instead, try to welcome discomfort as if to say to the pain, "I know you're going to do what you're going to do, but remember that we're all in this together, and you're not the enemy."

Whenever thoughts and emotions relating to the physical symptoms arise, relate to them in the same way you're relating to the physical symptoms themselves—notice them, feel them, and extend a healing awareness toward them.

Do your best to stay out of the mind that wants to analyze or blame, and instead keep the awareness centered in the chest and on the breath.

Continue to breathe into the center of the chest on the in-breath, and extend awareness to the place of discomfort on the out-breath, letting whatever arises just be.

Cultivating this attitude of warmth and receptivity, along with the movement of awareness-energy from the heart to the distress, is what heals. Particularly, extending awareness from the heart to our deepest pain, both physical and emotional, is a crucial step in learning to actually live from Being Kindness.

The real fruit of the practice life is not just about feeling better, nor is it just about having clarity. These things may certainly be included, but the real healing in our spiritual journey is the transformation out of the self-centered life of I-as-a-me. As we come to know the truth of who we really are—that the nature of our being is connectedness and love—we learn to live increasingly from the Zen Heart. Living from Being Kindness gradually becomes our natural response to life, even in the midst of our all-too-human pain. Our self-judgments of unworthiness and our conditioned fears may not completely disappear, but they no longer dictate who we are or how we live. The lightness of living from the awakened Heart makes possible a life of increasing joy and appreciation.

Appendix 1

The Essential Reminders

EACH OF THE FOLLOWING APHORISMS points to a key point in practice; taken together they serve as a summary of the main practices described in this book. One very helpful way to use these reminders is to pick one each day, returning to it repeatedly to remind yourself of what is most important.

- Remember your aspiration; without it there will only be sleep.

- Perseverance is the key, not how you feel.

- Don't try to change, just be aware.

- The fundamental question: Can I reside in my experience right now?

- Say yes to difficulties; they are not obstacles on the path; they *are* the path.

- Drop the story line of "me."

- Cultivate mercy toward yourself; compassion toward others will follow.

- Be present as often as possible; stay there as long as possible.

- The cardinal rule in relationships: refrain from blaming.

- Until you become intimate with your fears, they will always limit your ability to love.

- Residing in the Heart—not thinking, not doing, just Being.

- When you really pay attention, *everything* is your teacher.

- In this very moment, what would it mean to live from Being Kindness?

Appendix 2
Basic Meditation Instructions

IF POSSIBLE, it is best to sit (meditate) in the same place every day. The space should be uncluttered and conducive to quiet.

It is also helpful to sit at the same time every day—this will help foster the discipline necessary to overcome occasional laziness or loss of motivation to meditate.

Many find it helpful to have a small altar near where they sit. Lighting a candle or a stick of incense can help kindle your aspiration, as can having an inspirational picture or quotation on the altar.

Ideally, you would sit every day. At the very least, sit three to four times a week. When you first begin your meditation practice, it is okay to sit for just fifteen minutes, but you should gradually increase your time up to thirty to forty minutes.

Whether you sit on a cushion or a chair, it is important to sit in an erect but relaxed posture. Staying erect helps keep the mind alert; staying relaxed helps prevent unnecessary strain.

The eyes should be open, but looking down slightly. It is best to use "soft" eyes, or peripheral vision, where you're not looking directly at any particular point. The reason the eyes are kept open is that it is too easy to enter into a dreamy state with the eyes closed; this may admittedly feel pleasant, but closing your eyes is not conducive to being awake and aware, which is one of the main points of meditating.

Start by taking a couple of deep breaths in order to bring awareness into the body.

Then, to help settle the body and mind, bring a focused attention to the breath. Feel the specific physical sensations of the breath entering and leaving the body. For example, you can focus on the coolness of the breath as it enters the nostrils, and the subtle texture of the out-breath. Stay present with the physical experience of breathing for as long as you can, being aware of the tendency to have the attention pulled away into thinking, daydreaming, or planning.

You may get pulled away into thinking hundreds of times during a single sitting period. This is very normal, and there is no need to judge yourself as a bad meditator. Instead, each and every time you catch yourself lost in the mind, simply return to the physical sensations of the breath.

Many students find it helpful to count the breaths as a further aid to a focused attention. The instruction is to silently count from one to ten, counting only on the exhalation. If you get to ten, or if you lose track of where you are, simply start over at one.

It is fine to follow or count the breaths for the entire sitting period in the early stages, but if the mind and body begin to feel settled, it is good to let the awareness expand to include other sensations in the body, as well as input from the environment, such as sounds and the texture of the air. This allows you to move from a very concentrated awareness on just the breath to a more open state of awareness. Thoughts will no doubt continue to arise; the instruction is to notice them and then quickly turn away from the mental and back to awareness of physical reality.

Students often judge meditation periods as "bad" if they can't focus, or if they don't feel "good." But one of the great benefits of meditation comes from persevering anyway, regardless of how we feel. Eventually, a learning and a settling will begin to take place. And gradually, the sense of presence and equanimity that is cultivated through a daily meditation practice begins to be infused into our everyday living.

Appendix 3

The Three Vows

AT ZEN CENTER SAN DIEGO we do three full bows after periods of meditation, and with each bow I silently say one of the following lines. Each line corresponds to a stage in practice: the first line refers to the Me Phase; the second line refers to the phase of Being Awareness; and the third line refers to the phase of living from Being Kindness. They are each reminders to stay in touch with what is most important.

May I say yes to everything,
Going to the roots of fear.

May I be aware without ceasing,
Letting life just be.

May I see the face of God in everyone and everything,
Living from the heart of Being Kindness.

If you don't have a bowing practice, you can simply recite your vows before you begin meditating. If you light a candle or incense before sitting, that is an excellent time to repeat your vows, to remind yourself of the bigger picture of what you're doing. You don't have to use the three vows stated here; it's best to use words that are personally meaningful to you.

What is important is that you understand the need to work in all three phases of the practice life. Using specific vows helps to keep us focused on what we're actually doing in the three inter-penetrating phases.

Also by Ezra Bayda

Being Zen: Bringing Meditation to Life (Shambhala, 2002)

We can use whatever life presents, Ezra Bayda teaches, to strengthen our spiritual practice—including the turmoil of daily life. What we need is the willingness to just be with our experiences—whether they are painful or pleasing—opening ourselves to the reality of our lives without trying to fix or change anything. But doing this requires that we confront our most deeply rooted fears and assumptions in order to gradually become free of the constrictions and suffering they create. Then we can awaken to the loving-kindness that is at the heart of our being.

At Home in the Muddy Water: A Guide to Finding Peace within Everyday Chaos (Shambhala, 2004)

In this book, Bayda applies the simple Zen teaching of being "at home in the muddy water" to a range of everyday concerns—including relationships, trust, sexuality, and money—showing that everything we need to practice is right here before us, and that peace and fulfillment is available to everyone, right here, right now, no matter what their circumstances.

Saying Yes to Life (Even the Hard Parts) (Wisdom, 2005)

The teachings in *Saying Yes to Life* are presented in the form of brief aphorisms and one-page essays. Told in simple language, they provide inspiration for each day by stressing the importance of drawing meaning from life's paradoxes—opening to the unwanted, recognizing the possibility of equanimity within difficulty, and living for now rather than later.